Letting Go, Holding On

A Caregiver's Journey Through Dementia

By Sheri Rettew

Medical / Legal Disclaimer

This book is intended for informational and educational purposes only. It is not a substitute for professional medical, legal, or financial advice.

Dementia affects individuals differently, and the information in this book reflects general experiences and considerations, not individualized guidance. Always seek the advice of qualified healthcare providers regarding diagnosis, treatment, medications, or medical decisions.

Legal and financial information shared in this book is provided for general awareness only and should not be relied upon as legal or financial advice. Laws, regulations, and benefits vary by location and individual circumstances. Consult a qualified attorney, financial advisor, or appropriate professional for guidance specific to your situation.

While care has been taken to ensure the information in this book is accurate and compassionate, the author makes no guarantees regarding outcomes and assumes no responsibility for decisions made based on the content.

By reading this book, you acknowledge that caregiving decisions are complex and personal, and that responsibility for those decisions remains with you and your chosen professionals.

Table of Contents

If You Need Help Right Now

If you picked up this book because everything feels like too much right now, pause for a moment and breathe. Feeling overwhelmed in this situation is not a sign that you're failing—it's a sign that what you're carrying is incredibly heavy.

When you're in crisis, you do not need to read this book in order. Go straight to what matches your situation right now.

- **If you just received a diagnosis, or you're afraid one is coming**, go to **Chapter 1: When Dementia Is First Suspected** and **Chapter 2: The Diagnostic Process** for what to expect and what to do next.
- **If daily life at home feels unmanageable**, go to **Chapter 3: Learning to Communicate in a New Way** and **Chapter 4: Daily Caregiving Realities at Home** for practical approaches, scripts, and safety basics.
- **If you are emotionally exhausted, angry, guilty, or numb**, go to **Chapter 5: The Caregiver's Emotional World**, including the section *"If You're Feeling Overwhelmed or Unsafe,"* for validation and specific support resources.
- **If you're facing big decisions about placement**, go to **Chapter 8: Considering Memory Care or Skilled Facilities** and **Chapter 9: Life in a Facility** for guidance, decision tools, and checklists.
- **If you're worried about end of life or hospice**, go to **Chapter 10: The Final Stages and End of Life** for what to expect and how to think about "doing enough."

If at any point you feel unsafe, hopeless, or afraid of what you might do:

- In the United States, you can call or text **988** to reach the Suicide & Crisis Lifeline, available 24/7.
- Outside the U.S., look up your country's crisis line through national or local health services. Hospitals and emergency services can also help connect you to immediate support in most places.
- For dementia-specific emotional support and information, you can contact the **Alzheimer's Association** at **www.alz.org**, which offers a 24/7 helpline and caregiver resources.

Needing this kind of help does not mean you are weak or doing something wrong. It means your nervous system has reached its limit in an already impossible situation—and you deserve care, too.

Introduction

Loving Someone Through Dementia

I didn't understand what was happening at first. It felt like Tim Burton[1] had designed a merry-go-round, and I didn't want to ride it.

There wasn't a single moment when everything suddenly changed. Instead, it came quietly—small things that were easy to dismiss. A story repeated one too many times. A bill forgotten. A shift in personality that felt "off" but hard to explain. Like many families, we told ourselves it was part of the normal aging process, stress, or just a rough patch. Dementia wasn't the word we were ready to say out loud.

But once it enters your life, nothing is ever the same.

Caring for someone with dementia is not a straight path. It's not a before-and-after story. It's a long road of constant adjustment, where loss happens in pieces. You grieve while the person you love is still alive. You grieve who they were, the future you expected, the conversations you thought you'd still have, and the memories that now live only in you.

---

[1] Tim Burton (b. 1958) is an American filmmaker and artist renowned for his "Burtonesque" aesthetic, which blends gothic horror, German Expressionism, and dark whimsy. He is best known for directing cult classics such as *Beetlejuice* (1988), *Edward Scissorhands* (1990), and the 2022 hit series *Wednesday*. His work frequently explores the "sympathetic outcast" through high-contrast visuals and collaborations with composer Danny Elfman. For a look into his visual evolution, browse the Official Tim Burton Art Collection.

This book exists because dementia doesn't just affect the person diagnosed—it reshapes entire families. It challenges marriages, siblings, finances, identities, and mental health. It forces caregivers to make impossible decisions, often without guidance, validation, or support. And too often, it leaves people feeling isolated, guilty, and unsure if they're doing "enough."

I've been there.

I've lived the exhaustion of constant vigilance. The fear of medical emergencies. The heartbreak of watching someone fade while still breathing. I've felt the guilt that comes with resentment, the shame of wishing for rest, and the loneliness of realizing that very few people truly understand what this journey looks like from the inside.

What I learned—slowly, painfully, and often the hard way—is that dementia caregiving is not about fixing what cannot be fixed. It's about learning how to respond differently. How to advocate when your loved one can't. How to communicate when language no longer works the way it used to. How to find moments of meaning in the middle of loss.

This book is not here to sugarcoat dementia. It won't pretend that love alone makes it easier, or that there are perfect answers. What it will do is walk with you—step by step—from the moment dementia is suspected, through diagnosis, daily caregiving, difficult behaviors, financial and care decisions, placement in facilities when needed, and ultimately, through the end of life and the grief that follows.

You'll find practical guidance, yes—but also permission. Permission to grieve. Permission to feel overwhelmed.

Permission to ask for help. Permission to recognize that doing your best does not mean doing everything.

Most importantly, I want you to know this:

You are not failing. You are responding to an impossible situation with love.

Meaning isn't something we find in this journey. It's what we give to it—through love, strength, patience, advocacy, presence, and compassion, even when it hurts.

If you're holding this book because you're scared, exhausted, or unsure of what comes next, you're in the right place. You don't have to read it all at once. You don't have to have everything figured out. Just take the next step.

Why *"Letting Go, Holding On"*

I chose the title *"Letting Go, Holding On"* because that is what dementia caregiving asks of us, over and over again.

You are constantly letting go of who your loved one used to be, of the future you imagined, of conversations, roles, and expectations that no longer fit. You let go of certainty. You let go of control. You also grieve the shared memories you built together, and the feelings that lived inside those memories — joy, comfort, familiarity — now carried mostly by you alone. Eventually, you let go of pieces of yourself you didn't know were tied so tightly to this relationship.

And at the same time, you are holding on.

You hold on to love, even when recognition fades. You hold on to dignity when independence slips away. You hold on to routines, small moments, fragments of connection, and the responsibility to keep showing up — even when the road keeps changing beneath your feet.

Dementia caregiving is not a clean transition from one role to another. It is an emotional push-and-pull that exists all at once. Letting go does not mean giving up. Holding on does not mean refusing reality.

Most days, you are doing both — often in the same moment.

This book is meant to sit with you in that tension, not try to resolve it. There is no single moment when you fully release one role and step cleanly into another. There is only the ongoing work of adjusting, grieving, loving, and responding to what is in front of you now.

That is the space this book lives in.

Let's begin.

How to Use This Book

If you're reading this in a moment of crisis, take a breath first.

This book is not meant to be read straight through, although it can be and will become an important part of your caregiving toolkit, I hope. It's not a test you need to pass. Dementia caregiving doesn't happen in order, and neither does learning how to survive it. You may be here because something just happened—a fall, a diagnosis, an argument, a sudden decline, or a decision you never wanted to make.

That's okay.

Use this book the way you need to. Skip ahead. Re-read sections. Put it down when it's too much. Some chapters may not apply to you yet; others may feel painfully familiar. You don't need to absorb everything at once.

If you're overwhelmed, start with the chapter that matches what you're facing *right now*.

If you're planning ahead, read slowly and come back when things change.

If you're grieving, know that what you're feeling is valid—even if your loved one is still alive.

This book is both practical and personal. It offers guidance, but it also offers permission: permission to rest, permission to hurt, to ask for help, to feel conflicted, and to make decisions without having all the answers.

There is no "right" way to do this. There is only the best you can do with the information, energy, and support you have at this moment.

You are not behind. You are not failing. You are responding to something incredibly hard.

Let this book be a companion—not a rulebook.

Read what you need. Leave the rest for later.

You're not alone.

Chapter 1 — When Dementia Is First Suspected

The earliest signs rarely arrive with sureness or clarity.

For me, they showed up as mild, infrequent panic attacks. My mom was in her mid-60s, driving on roads she had traveled for more than forty-five years—roads she could have driven with her eyes closed. Suddenly, she would pull over, call someone for reassurance, or abandon a trip altogether. I assumed it was anxiety. She had struggled with it in her 30s and 40s, and this felt like a familiar pattern resurfacing. It didn't alarm me. It didn't feel like the beginning of anything irreversible.

Looking back, that's how dementia often enters a family's life—quietly, plausibly, and wrapped in explanations that make sense at the time.

It wasn't until years later, when my mom was 75, that something shifted inside me. She didn't give me a birthday card. That may sound small, but it wasn't. My entire life, she had never missed it—not once. This time, there was no apology, no explanation, no sense that she even realized it mattered. She seemed almost disinterested.

I remember thinking, *Here we go. This is what it's going to feel like.*

My mom loved me fiercely as her only child. That love wasn't always healthy for either of us, but it was real and unwavering.

By then, her memory issues, mood changes, and cognitive function were no longer subtle. They were persistent enough that I couldn't explain them away anymore.

That's often the moment families reach—the one where instinct quietly overrides denial.

The Signs We Explain Away

When dementia is first suspected, it rarely looks like what people expect. It doesn't usually begin with forgetting names or not recognizing loved ones. Instead, it often shows up as:

- Changes in mood or personality
- Increased anxiety or panic
- Difficulty with familiar tasks
- Subtle judgment changes
- Withdrawal or loss of interest
- Trouble following conversations or plans

Because these changes are gradual, we tell ourselves stories to make them less frightening. *They're stressed. They're grieving. They're depressed. They're getting older.* Sometimes those explanations are true. Sometimes they aren't.

What makes this stage so difficult is that there's no single moment that demands action. Just a growing sense that something is off—and the discomfort of not knowing what to do with that feeling.

Cultural and Family Contexts in Dementia Care

Dementia does not exist in a vacuum. Cultural background, family structure, spiritual beliefs, and expectations around aging all influence how early changes are noticed, talked about, and responded to.

In some families or cultures, memory changes may be minimized out of respect for elders, fear of stigma, or a belief that decline is simply part of normal aging. In others, caregiving is viewed as a shared responsibility, while some caregivers may feel pressure—spoken or unspoken—to manage everything on their own. These differences can shape when help is sought, how decisions are made, and how much support a caregiver feels permitted to accept.

None of these approaches is inherently right or wrong. What matters most is safety, dignity, and support—for your loved one and for you. As you read this book, take what fits your values and circumstances, and leave what does not. Your cultural and family context matters, and it deserves respect.

What We Mean When We Say "Dementia"

Dementia isn't a single disease. It's a term used to describe a group of symptoms caused by changes in the brain that affect memory, thinking, behavior, and the ability to function independently.

People often think dementia means forgetting names or getting lost—but it's much more complex than that. It can affect judgment, emotions, personality, communication, and the ability to understand what's happening.

This is one reason dementia is so disorienting for families. The changes don't always look the way we expect.

Understanding Stages—Without a Timeline

You may hear dementia described in stages—early, middle, and late—or through clinical scales (stages 1-7). These frameworks can be helpful, but they can also be misleading if taken too literally.

Dementia does not progress neatly or predictably.

Someone may:

- Appear capable one day and confused the next
- Function well in familiar settings but struggle elsewhere
- Decline slowly in one area and rapidly in another

Staging focuses primarily on daily functioning—such as self-care and safety—rather than on memory scores alone. How someone manages daily life matters more than test scores.

If staging feels confusing, that's because it often is.

A Note About Comparison

It's natural to compare your loved one's experience to others. Try to be gentle with yourself and others when you do.

Dementia journeys vary widely depending on the type of dementia, overall health, personality, and support. Here's one of those 'A Caregiver's Voice' moments I mentioned in the introduction—an analogy to relate to complex ideas.

A Caregiver's Voice

I have been heavily involved in working with child sexual abuse as a public health crisis and working with victims' loved ones. Sometimes, I like to use what I call "Fisher-Price" analogies to help me understand complex ideas. I found this to be so helpful when explaining the "whys" that come up in that industry.

In this case, think about taste buds. Some people like coconut, for instance, and others can't stand it (I'm in the latter group in case you're interested). Everyone is different, a complex recipe of biology, upbringing, coping mechanisms, external support systems, and experiences. There is no "right" way—and no version that means you're missing something.

Understanding dementia doesn't require mastering every detail. It starts with recognizing that what you're seeing is real—and that you're not imagining it.

When Love Makes It Harder

It's especially complicated when the person experiencing these changes has always been deeply involved, loving, or emotionally expressive. When someone who once remembered every detail suddenly forgets something meaningful, it can feel personal—even when it isn't.

This is where guilt often begins. And grief.

You wonder if you're overreacting. You question whether you're being unfair. You worry about labeling something too soon. And when the person insists they're fine, the doubt grows stronger.

But dementia doesn't announce itself clearly. It whispers first.

Understanding What's Really Happening

One of the most important things to understand early on is that many people with dementia genuinely do not recognize the changes happening to them. This isn't denial in the emotional sense—it's neurological. The brain loses its ability to accurately self-assess.

This lack of awareness is called *anosognosia (a neurological lack of awareness of deficits)*, and it's one of the most frustrating aspects of the disease. Your loved one may insist nothing is wrong, become defensive when concerns are raised, or accuse others of exaggerating or interfering.

Knowing this early can help you stop arguing with facts that no longer land the way they once did.

How Stages Are Determined (and Why They Feel Vague)

Families often ask, *What stage are we in?* early on, hoping it will bring clarity or direction. While staging systems exist, dementia doesn't follow a predictable timeline. Progression varies widely depending on the type of dementia, overall health, and individual biology.

Providers often assess progression by looking at ADLs— Activities of Daily Living—rather than memory alone.

Stages are typically determined by function, not just memory. Doctors look at how well someone manages daily activities. You'll hear a lot about ADLs (activities of daily living in the early phases), decision-making, communication, and self-care—not just test scores.

This is why two people with the same diagnosis can look completely different.

A General Sense of How Dementia Often Progresses

While dementia doesn't follow a straight line, many caregivers find it helpful to have a *general* sense of how changes often unfold. This isn't a checklist, a timeline, or a prediction. It's simply a way to orient yourself when things start to feel unfamiliar.

Early Changes: The Stage We Explain Away

Early dementia is often subtle and inconsistent. Memory lapses come and go. Personality shifts are easy to rationalize. Everyone involved may sense that *something* is off, but not enough to name it confidently.

Caregivers often notice:

- Repeated stories or questions
- Increased anxiety or rigidity
- Trouble with planning, driving, or finances
- Subtle personality or mood changes

Emotionally, this stage is filled with doubt. Caregivers second-guess themselves, minimize concerns, or worry about overreacting. Many later realize this was the stage where intuition mattered most.

If you're here, trust that noticing doesn't mean labeling. It means paying attention.

Middle Changes: When Daily Life Is Affected

As dementia progresses, changes begin to interfere with daily functioning. Tasks that once felt automatic require support. Behavior may become unpredictable.

Caregivers often notice:

- Difficulty with personal care
- Communication breakdowns
- Agitation, anxiety, or withdrawal
- Safety concerns

- Resistance to help

This is often the most demanding stage for caregivers. You may feel stretched thin, constantly adjusting, and unsure which version of your loved one you'll encounter each day.

Needing help during this stage is not a sign of failure. It's a response to increasing complexity.

Later Changes: When the Body Slows Down

In later stages, physical decline becomes more visible. Dependence increases. Communication fades.

Caregivers often notice:

- Limited mobility
- Increased sleeping
- Difficulty eating or swallowing
- Minimal verbal response

This stage can feel like a prolonged goodbye. Grief is often present even before death occurs. (More later on this.)

Understanding these stages doesn't make them easier — but it can help you recognize that what you're seeing is part of the disease, not something you caused.

Quick Home Safety Checklist

You do not have to do all of this at once; start where risk feels highest. You don't need to make your home feel like a medical facility. Small, thoughtful changes can reduce risk and ease stress—for both you and your loved one.

You don't have to do everything at once. Start where it feels most urgent.

Basic Home Safety

- Improve lighting, especially in hallways, bathrooms, and near stairs
- Reduce clutter and remove loose rugs or cords that could cause falls
- Install grab bars in bathrooms and consider non-slip mats in tubs and showers
- Make stairs safer with handrails on both sides and clear visual edges
- Install wireless cameras if you must leave your loved one alone, as a precaution.

Exits and Wandering Safety

- Secure doors discreetly if wandering becomes a concern (alarms, chimes, or visual barriers)
- Keep keys and exit points consistent to reduce confusion
- Consider an ID bracelet or card with name and contact information, especially if wandering risk increases

Medication Safety

- Store medications securely and out of sight
- Use a pill organizer filled by one designated person
- Keep a written medication list to avoid duplicate dosing. This will also come in handy at doctor appointments.
- Watch for confusion around "already taken" versus "not yet taken."

Driving Safety

Changes in driving ability often appear earlier than expected and can be hard to talk about.

Watch for:

- Getting lost on familiar routes
- Increased anxiety, panic, or confusion while driving
- New dents or scrapes on the car
- Slower reaction time or difficulty following traffic rules

If concerns arise:

- Limit driving gradually rather than abruptly, when possible
- Involve a healthcare provider to support the conversation
- Frame changes around safety and support—not punishment

Revisiting safety doesn't mean things are getting "worse."

It means you're responding to change with care.

Making Provisions for Pets

Pets are often deeply bonded to their owners, and changes in routine or ability can affect both the person with dementia and the animal. Early planning can prevent unnecessary stress later.

Consider:

- Who can help with feeding, walking, or veterinary care if abilities change

- Whether the pet could safely remain in the home
- Long-term plans if your loved one moves to a facility
- Including pet care wishes in legal or family planning conversations

Planning for pets isn't just practical—it's compassionate. It protects a relationship that often brings comfort when so much else feels uncertain.

Start Documenting—Even If You're Not Ready

If there is one practical step that helps at this stage, it's documentation. Keep a simple log of incidents, questions, and patterns; it will be invaluable during later medical appointments.

Not because you're committing to a diagnosis—but because patterns matter.

Start writing things down:

- Dates and descriptions of concerning behaviors
- Medical issues or sudden changes
- Incidents while driving or navigating familiar places
- Emotional shifts or personality changes

This record becomes invaluable later—for doctors, for care planning, and for your own clarity when doubt creeps in.

I highly recommend keeping a journal, even if you haven't before. Nothing fancy is required–a spiral notebook works just fine. You may find it even helps with documenting and advocating for your loved one.

Create a Central Information Hub

As you begin documenting changes — dates, behaviors, conversations — there is another step that may not feel urgent yet, but will become invaluable later.

Gather the practical pieces of your loved one's life into one organized place. This will help you immeasurably, even if dementia is not the diagnosis. It becomes an invaluable resource over time — supporting medical appointments, financial decisions, and any level of care that may eventually be needed.

In the early stages of dementia, people often still manage their own accounts, appointments, and paperwork. But subtle shifts can happen quickly. Passwords are forgotten. Bills are misplaced. Medical histories become harder to recall. And when decisions need to be made, the stress of searching for information can compound an already emotional moment.

Creating one central location for essential information is not about assuming the worst. It's about reducing chaos if and when things become complicated.

This can be a binder, a notebook, a digital file system, or a combination of both. Some families call it "Our Portfolio." Others simply label it "Important Documents." The title doesn't matter. Consistency does.

Having everything accessible in one place will save time, prevent unnecessary panic, and allow you to advocate more effectively when the time comes.

What to Include

Start with what you can access now. You do not need to gather everything in a single afternoon.

Consider including:

- Copies of legal documents (Power of Attorney, healthcare directives, wills, trusts)
- Insurance policies and contact information
- Social Security, Medicare, and pension details
- Bank accounts and financial institutions
- Investment or retirement accounts
- List of medications and prescribing physicians
- Primary care provider and specialist contact information
- Account numbers and customer service phone numbers
- Email addresses and usernames
- A secure password management plan
- Safe deposit box location and key information
- Funeral or end-of-life preferences, if discussed

If possible:

- Keep a copy in a fireproof safe.
- Share access details with one trusted secondary person.
- Review and update the information every few months.

Organization will not change the diagnosis.

But it will reduce future scrambling and protect you from making decisions under pressure without the information you need.

Think of this as creating a small anchor point — something steady to hold onto when the rest of the journey begins to shift.

Giving Meaning to the Beginning

This early stage is often filled with uncertainty and second-guessing. It's also where caregivers begin to quietly change—learning to observe, to adapt, and to protect without yet knowing how far the road goes.

Meaning doesn't come from certainty here. It comes from attention. From noticing. From caring enough to ask hard questions before answers are available.

If you're at this point—uneasy, uncertain, and not ready to name what's happening—know that this is a valid place to be. You don't need to have it all figured out.

You only need to pay attention.

The next step, when you're ready, is understanding how concern becomes diagnosis—and how to navigate that process without losing yourself or your loved one in the system.

That's where we'll go next.

Reflection Prompts

You don't need to answer every question. Choose the ones that feel useful right now.

- What were the first changes I noticed that made me pause, even if I explained them away at the time?
- Are there moments that felt "small" then but now seem meaningful when I look back?
- What explanations have I been using to make sense of what's happening, and how do they make me feel?

- What emotions come up when I consider that something more serious may be going on?
- Am I feeling pressure—from myself or others—to be certain before I'm ready?
- What would it look like to simply observe right now, without trying to fix or label anything?
- Who could I talk to about my concerns without feeling judged or dismissed?

A Gentle Reminder

It's okay if you don't have answers yet.

It's okay if your feelings are mixed or contradictory.

Awareness is not the same as acceptance—and you're allowed to move at your own pace.

Chapter 2 — The Diagnostic Process

For many families, the decision to pursue a diagnosis doesn't come from certainty. It comes from the desire to disprove that the diagnosis is dementia. Or it comes from accumulation.

It's the growing stack of moments you can no longer ignore. The uneasy feeling that keeps returning. The quiet realization that waiting for things to "go back to normal" isn't working anymore.

Seeking a diagnosis doesn't mean you're ready for answers. It simply means you're ready for clarity—whatever that clarity turns out to be.

Understanding Different Forms of Dementia

"Dementia" is not a single disease—it's an umbrella term. Alzheimer's disease is the most widely known, but there are many forms, including vascular dementia, Lewy body dementia, frontotemporal dementia, and mixed dementias.

Each affects the brain differently, which is why symptoms vary so much. Some people experience memory loss early. Others struggle first with language, judgment, movement, or behavior.

This variability is one reason comparisons can be misleading. Your loved one's journey may look very different from someone else's—and that doesn't mean you're misunderstanding what's happening.

When Concern Becomes Action

People often worry that asking for an evaluation is a betrayal or that it will permanently label their loved one before they're ready. But the diagnostic process is not a single test or a single appointment. It's a series of observations, conversations, and rule-outs.

At this stage, many caregivers feel caught between two fears:

- *What if something is really wrong?*
- *What if nothing is—and I've overreacted?*

Both fears can exist at the same time.

The goal of diagnosis isn't to rush to dementia—it's to understand what's happening and why. Memory loss and cognitive changes can come from many sources, some of them are treatable. That's why this step matters.

What the Diagnostic Process Usually Involves

While every experience is different, a dementia evaluation often includes some combination of:

- A detailed medical history
- Cognitive and memory testing
- Neurological exams
- Blood work to rule out deficiencies or infections
- Brain imaging (CT, MRI, or PET scans in some cases)

This process can take time. Appointments may feel fragmented. Results may be inconclusive at first. And the waiting is horrible.

Waiting for referrals, waiting for results, waiting, waiting, waiting. That uncertainty can be frustrating—but it's common.

It's also common for caregivers to notice changes long before test results clearly reflect them. Trust your observations. You live with the person. You see what clinicians don't.

Many caregivers are surprised to learn that dementia care rarely happens inside a single, coordinated system—medical, legal, financial, and caregiving supports often exist separately, and part of the caregiver's role is connecting the dots.

Is Dementia Hereditary?

This is one of the most common—and emotionally charged—questions caregivers ask.

The short answer is: sometimes, but often not in a simple or predictable way.

Most cases of dementia are not directly inherited. Having a parent or close relative with dementia does not mean you will develop it. Some genetic factors can increase risk, particularly in Alzheimer's disease, but they are only part of a much larger picture that includes age, overall health, lifestyle, and environmental factors.

Rare forms of dementia are strongly genetic, but these are uncommon and usually appear earlier in life.

If you're worried about your own risk, a healthcare provider or genetic counselor can help you understand what—if any—family history information is relevant. For many caregivers, reassurance and monitoring are far more appropriate than testing.

This keeps fear from spiraling.

Quick Guide: When to Call the Doctor (and When It Can Wait)

Not every change is an emergency—but some changes should never be ignored.

Consider calling the doctor promptly if you notice:

- Sudden or dramatic changes in behavior or alertness
- New or worsening confusion over hours or days
- Signs of pain your loved one can't explain
- Fever, burning with urination, or foul-smelling urine (possible UTI)
- Falls, especially with head injury
- New difficulty swallowing or choking

Changes that can often be monitored (but still noted):

- Gradual memory decline
- Mild changes in sleep patterns
- Occasional agitation that resolves with reassurance

If something feels different or alarming to you, trust that instinct. You know your loved one better than anyone else.

Doctor Visit Worksheet: Making the Most of Each Appointment

Not every change is an emergency—but some changes should never be ignored. You are not expected to sort this out alone; this guide is meant to give you a starting point when you're unsure. You don't need to bring perfect notes. A simple page can make appointments less overwhelming and help your providers see what you see.

Before the appointment

- ☐ Top 3 changes I've noticed since the last visit (memory, behavior, safety, mood):
- ☐ Medications and doses (including over-the-counter and supplements):
- ☐ Name / dose / how often
- ☐ Any side effects or concerns
- ☐ Specific questions I want to ask:
- ☐ About diagnosis (what do you think is happening and why?)
- ☐ About safety (driving, falls, living alone)
- ☐ About medications (what they can and cannot do, side effects to watch for)

During the appointment

Take a notebook or notepad, or use the notes app on your phone. It's important to document what is said so you can refer to it later.

☐   What the provider said is most likely going on:

☐   Tests or referrals they ordered (and why):

☐   Any changes to medications or safety
recommendations:

After the appointment

☐   What still feels unclear to me:

☐   What I need to watch for at home or track for the next
visit:

Common Medical Issues That Complicate Dementia

Even early in the disease process, people with cognitive
impairment are more vulnerable to certain medical problems
that can worsen symptoms suddenly.

Urinary tract infections (UTIs), dehydration, electrolyte
imbalances, and infections can cause dramatic changes in
behavior, confusion, or agitation—sometimes almost overnight.
These episodes can be terrifying if you don't know what's
happening.

A sudden decline does not always mean rapid progression of
dementia. Sometimes it means something else is wrong—and
treatable. This is why medical evaluation remains important
throughout the journey.

Quick Guide: When Things Change Suddenly

A sudden change in behavior, confusion, agitation, or physical ability can be frightening. It's natural to assume the dementia has rapidly worsened—but sudden changes are often caused by something else, and many are treatable.

Before assuming this is dementia progression, consider common triggers:

- Urinary tract infections (UTIs) — especially common in older adults and often present without typical symptoms
- Dehydration
- Pain (including pain your loved one cannot clearly express)
- Medication changes, missed doses, or side effects
- Constipation
- Infections (respiratory, dental, skin)
- Sleep disruption or extreme fatigue

What to do next:

- Trust your instinct if something feels "off."
- Contact your loved one's primary care provider or neurologist and describe the change clearly and specifically.
- Ask whether lab work or a medical evaluation is appropriate before assuming cognitive decline.
- If symptoms are severe, sudden, or involve safety concerns, seek urgent or emergency care.

Sudden changes are stressful—but they are also a signal to pause, assess, and advocate, not to panic or assume the worst.

Many caregivers discover that addressing the underlying issue brings meaningful improvement.

Understanding Sundowning

Many caregivers notice a confusing pattern early on: their loved one seems relatively stable during part of the day, only to become more anxious, agitated, confused, or emotional as evening approaches.

This pattern is commonly called **sundowning**.

Sundowning is not a separate diagnosis. It's a term used to describe a cluster of symptoms that tend to worsen in the late afternoon or evening in people with dementia.

These symptoms may include:

- Increased confusion or disorientation
- Anxiety or restlessness
- Agitation or irritability
- Suspicion or paranoia
- Emotional outbursts
- Difficulty settling down for the night

For caregivers, sundowning can feel abrupt and alarming—especially when it happens for the first time. It can also be exhausting, especially when caregivers are already tired themselves.

For more on evening behavior and safety, see Chapter 4 (Daily Realities) and Chapter 8 (Considering In-Home Care, Memory Care...).

Why Sundowning Happens

There isn't a single cause of sundowning, but several factors may contribute:

- Fatigue from a full day of stimulation
- Changes in lighting that increase confusion
- Disruption of circadian rhythms
- Hunger, thirst, or pain that's difficult to express
- Sensory overload or under-stimulation

Sundowning does **not** mean dementia has suddenly worsened. It reflects how the brain struggles with transitions, fatigue, and sensory processing.

What Caregivers Should Know Early

Not every person with dementia experiences sundowning, and its severity can vary widely. For some, it's mild. For others, it becomes one of the most challenging parts of the day.

Importantly, sundowning does not automatically require medication. Many non-drug strategies—routine, calm environments, gentle reassurance, and physical needs being met—can reduce its impact. Medications are sometimes considered when symptoms cause significant distress or safety concerns, but they are not the first or only option.

Understanding sundowning early helps caregivers respond with compassion rather than panic.

Common Medications Used in Dementia Care: What Caregivers Should Know

When medications enter the picture, many caregivers feel a mix of hope and fear. Hope that something might help. Fear of side effects, personality changes, or making the wrong decision.

Medications are listed so you can become familiar with possibilities. But every person is an individual and may have other health issues, so it's important to talk to your loved one's doctors if you are wondering whether a medication will help.

It's important to know this up front: medications for dementia are about symptom management, not curative. They are tools that may help with memory, mood, anxiety, sleep, or behavior—but they work differently for each person, and benefits are often modest.

That doesn't mean they're meaningless, but I want you to have clear expectations. Many medications used in dementia care are prescribed to manage symptoms rather than the disease itself, and each comes with potential benefits and risks.

Below are some of the most commonly prescribed medications caregivers encounter, along with their common uses. It can be uncomfortable to introduce some of these medications to your loved one, particularly if they've never needed them in the past.

A Caregiver's Voice

Another of my Fisher-Price analogies. Think of a diabetic or someone with cancer. They need insulin or other medications or treatments to live the healthiest life possible. Medication should be looked at as a tool to help your loved one experience peace and comfort.

Medications Aimed at Memory and Cognition

Donepezil (Aricept)

Aricept is one of the most commonly prescribed medications for Alzheimer's disease and other dementias.

- **What it's used for:**
  Memory, attention, and thinking skills—primarily in early to moderate stages

- **What it may help:**
  Some people experience slower cognitive decline or improved alertness.

- **Common side effects:**
  Nausea, diarrhea, appetite loss, vivid dreams, and sleep disturbances

Not everyone benefits from Aricept, and some people cannot tolerate the side effects. A lack of improvement does not mean the medication "failed"—it may simply not be a good match for that individual.

Other medications in this same category include rivastigmine (Exelon) and galantamine.

Memantine (Namenda)

Memantine is often prescribed for moderate to later stages of dementia and works differently from medications like donepezil (Aricept). It may help with cognition, daily functioning, or behavioral symptoms for some individuals.

Effects vary widely. Some caregivers notice modest stabilization; others see little change. As with all dementia medications, benefits must be weighed against side effects.

Monoclonal Antibodies

Newer medications known as monoclonal antibodies have been developed to target specific proteins associated with Alzheimer's disease. These treatments are typically offered only to individuals in very early stages and under strict eligibility criteria.

They require frequent monitoring and carry potential risks, including brain swelling or bleeding. For many families, these medications are not appropriate or accessible. Discuss risks, benefits, and expectations thoroughly with a specialist before pursuing this option.

Medications for Agitation, Aggression, or Severe Behavioral Symptoms

Gabapentin

Gabapentin is sometimes used to help manage anxiety, agitation, nerve pain, or restlessness in people with dementia. It may also support sleep in some cases.

Like many medications used off-label in dementia care, responses vary. Drowsiness and balance issues can occur, so monitoring is important.

Quetiapine (Seroquel)

Quetiapine is an antipsychotic medication sometimes used to help manage severe agitation, aggression, hallucinations, or distress that has not responded to other approaches. It is often considered when safety or quality of life is at risk.

Antipsychotics carry important risks for people with dementia, including increased risk of falls, sedation, and, in some cases, serious cardiovascular events. Because of this, they are typically used at the lowest effective dose and reassessed frequently.

For some families, quetiapine provides meaningful relief from intense distress. For others, side effects outweigh benefits. Clear communication with providers about goals, risks, and monitoring is essential.

Risperidone (Risperdal)

Risperidone is an antipsychotic medication sometimes used when behaviors become unsafe or extremely distressing.

- **What it's used for:**
  Severe agitation, aggression, paranoia, or hallucinations

- **When it's considered:**
  Usually, after non-medication strategies have failed

- **Important considerations:**
  Antipsychotics carry significant risks in older adults with dementia, including increased risk of stroke and death.

These medications are often prescribed with caution and should be regularly re-evaluated. If your loved one is prescribed an antipsychotic, it's reasonable—and important—to ask why, for how long, and how success will be measured.

Medications for Anxiety and Acute Distress

Lorazepam (Ativan)

Ativan is a benzodiazepine used for short-term anxiety or panic.

- **What it's used for:**
  Acute anxiety, panic attacks, medical procedures, or extreme distress

- **What caregivers may notice:**
  Sedation, increased confusion, or unsteadiness

- **Important caution:**
  Benzodiazepines can worsen confusion and increase fall risk, especially with regular use.

While Ativan can be helpful in specific situations, long-term or frequent use can sometimes make symptoms worse rather than better.

Antidepressants

Antidepressants are commonly used in dementia care—not just for depression, but also for anxiety, irritability, and emotional regulation.

- **What they're used for:**
  Depression, anxiety, mood instability, tearfulness, withdrawal

- **Common classes:**
  SSRIs such as sertraline (Zoloft), citalopram (Celexa), or

escitalopram (Lexapro)

- **Why they're often chosen:**
  Generally safer than antipsychotics for long-term use

Caregivers sometimes notice improved mood, reduced irritability, or better sleep—but changes can take weeks, not days.

Medications for Pain

Acetaminophen (Tylenol Extra Strength)

Pain in people with dementia is often underrecognized because it may not be expressed clearly. Acetaminophen is commonly used to address chronic or unexplained discomfort that may be contributing to agitation or behavior changes.

Even over-the-counter medications should be used intentionally and monitored, especially when taken regularly.

Tramadol

Tramadol is an opioid pain medication sometimes prescribed for moderate pain when other options are insufficient. Pain in people with dementia is often underrecognized, and untreated pain can contribute to agitation, restlessness, or behavior changes.

Tramadol can cause side effects such as confusion, sedation, dizziness, or increased fall risk—particularly in older adults or those with cognitive impairment. It may also interact with other medications commonly used in dementia care.

When tramadol is prescribed, caregivers should watch closely for changes in alertness, balance, or behavior and report concerns promptly. Pain relief should always be balanced with safety and overall comfort.

Medications for Sleep and Sundowning

Sleep disturbances are common in dementia, particularly as circadian rhythms change and sundowning becomes more pronounced. Difficulty falling asleep, nighttime waking, or increased evening agitation can be exhausting for both the person with dementia and their caregiver.

Because of this, sleep medications are sometimes suggested—but they are prescribed cautiously.

Some medications may help regulate sleep-wake cycles or reduce nighttime distress. Others, however, can increase confusion, worsen balance, or cause excessive daytime sleepiness.

Whenever sleep medications are suggested, it's reasonable to ask whether non-drug strategies can be tried first. Throughout my own loved one's journey, one of my greatest concerns was not wanting to sedate her for the entire day just to make the night easier.

A Caregiver's Voice

When sleep medications were suggested for my loved one, my biggest fear wasn't the night—it was the day that might disappear afterward. I didn't want her to be "out of it," or asleep, if it meant she was no longer present. That concern shaped many of my decisions, and it's okay if it shapes yours, too.

That concern is valid.

Sedation can reduce nighttime symptoms, but it can also take away meaningful waking hours, increase fall risk, and dull engagement. For many caregivers, the goal isn't simply sleep—it's preserving quality of life, alertness, and dignity as much as possible.

If sleep medications are used, they should be revisited regularly. What helps at one stage may become harmful at another.

What Medications Cannot Do

This is one of the hardest truths to accept.

Medications cannot:

- Restore lost memories
- Stop disease progression
- Bring back the person your loved one used to be

If a medication seems to help, it may be subtle: fewer distressing behaviors, slightly better focus, or a calmer emotional baseline.

Small improvements matter—but so does quality of life.

Your Role as a Medication Advocate

Caregivers are often the first to notice side effects, changes, or problems. You don't need medical training to notice when something doesn't feel right.

Keep notes on:

- When medications are started, stopped, or adjusted
- Changes in behavior, sleep, appetite, or mobility
- New confusion or worsening symptoms

Ask questions like:

- *What symptom is this medication meant to help?*
- *How will we know if it's working?*
- *What side effects should I watch for?*
- *Is this medication intended to be short-term or ongoing?*

You are allowed to revisit decisions. Medication plans should evolve as the disease changes.

A Gentle Perspective

Medication decisions are rarely clear-cut. Sometimes they help. Sometimes they don't. Sometimes the "right" choice changes over time.

There is no perfect answer—only informed, compassionate decisions made with the information available at the moment.

And that is enough.

Advocating During the Diagnostic Process

This stage often introduces caregivers to a new role: that of an advocate.

You may find yourself translating behaviors into clinical language, correcting misunderstandings, or pushing for follow-up when something doesn't feel right. This can feel uncomfortable—especially if you're used to trusting authority figures.

But advocacy isn't about confrontation. It's about clarity.

Bring your documentation. Ask for explanations in plain language. Repeat concerns if needed. If something doesn't make sense, say so. You are not wasting anyone's time.

The Emotional Impact of Naming What's Happening

Receiving a diagnosis—or even a strong suspicion—can feel like grief and relief colliding.

Grief, because something has been named that cannot be undone.

Relief, because you're no longer imagining things.

Some caregivers feel numb. Others feel overwhelmed. Some feel validated. All of these responses are normal.

There is no requirement to feel a certain way.

You don't need to make every decision immediately. You don't need to tell everyone right away. You don't need to know what the rest of the journey will look like.

A diagnosis is not the end of hope—it's the beginning of informed care.

Reflection Prompts

You don't need to work through these all at once. Choose what feels relevant right now.

- ☐ What specific changes or moments finally made me consider asking for an evaluation?
- ☐ What fears or hopes do I carry into the diagnostic process?
- ☐ How do I feel when I imagine hearing the words "dementia" out loud?
- ☐ In what ways have I been doubting my own observations, and what helps me trust them more?
- ☐ What would I most want the doctor to understand about my loved one—not just their symptoms, but who they are?
- ☐ What support (practical or emotional) would make this stage feel more bearable?
- ☐ After each appointment, what do I want to notice about how I'm doing—not just how my loved one is doing?

A Gentle Reminder

Needing clarity does not mean you are giving up on hope.

Your day-to-day observations are real data. They matter just as much as test scores or scans.

If the process feels slow, fragmented, or confusing, that isn't a failure on your part. It's the nature of the system—and you're doing your best to navigate it.

Looking Ahead

Once dementia is suspected or diagnosed, the question often becomes: *How do I talk to them now?*

How do you explain appointments, changes, or concerns without causing fear or conflict? How do you preserve dignity when communication itself is changing?

That's where we're headed next—learning how to communicate in a way that reduces distress and protects connection, even as language and understanding begin to shift.

Chapter 3 — Learning to Communicate in a New Way

One of the hardest shifts in dementia caregiving is realizing that communication, as you've always known it, no longer works.

You may still be using the same words, the same tone, the same logic—but the response you get feels confusing, frustrating, or heartbreaking. Conversations that once felt easy now end in agitation, silence, or conflict. And often, both of you walk away feeling upset without fully understanding why.

This isn't because you're doing something wrong.

It's because dementia changes how the brain processes language, memory, reasoning, and emotion. Communication becomes less about exchanging information and more about creating a sense of safety.

What's Really Changing

As dementia progresses, the brain gradually loses the ability to:

- Process complex language
- Hold multiple pieces of information at once
- Recall recent events accurately
- Understand abstract ideas or time-based questions
- Filter emotions appropriately

This means that questions, explanations, or corrections that once made sense may now feel overwhelming, confusing, or threatening.

When communication breaks down, behavior often takes its place.

Agitation, withdrawal, repetition, anger, or tears are frequently expressions of unmet needs—not intentional behavior. Understanding this reframes communication from *getting the right answer* to *reducing distress*.

When Your Loved One Insists Nothing Is Wrong (Anosognosia)

This lack of awareness is neurological, not denial.

You might try:

- Avoiding debates about diagnosis
- Framing helps as convenience, not a necessity
- Adjusting the environment quietly rather than explaining changes

Insight cannot be forced. Safety can still be supported.

A Shift in Goal: From Accuracy to Comfort

One of the most painful adjustments caregivers make is letting go of the need for accuracy.

Correcting facts, reminding someone of what they've forgotten, or pointing out inconsistencies may feel logical—but for a person with dementia, it can feel humiliating or frightening. The brain is no longer able to reconcile those corrections, even when they are true.

The goal of communication becomes comfort, not correction.

There is usually nothing to be gained by arguing or trying to correct someone. They are unlikely to retain the information, and you're both frustrated. The goal becomes connection, not compliance.

How to Talk to Someone with Dementia

There is no script that works every time, but there *are* approaches that tend to reduce frustration for both of you.

Use simple, direct language

- Speak slowly and calmly
- Use short sentences
- Focus on one idea at a time

Avoid questions that require memory or decision-making

- Don't ask if they remember something
- Avoid multiple-choice questions
- Avoid open-ended questions like "What do you want to do today?"

A Caregiver's Voice: Meeting Them Where They Are

One of the most important communication lessons I've learned is this: **my mom can no longer meet me in my world — so I climb into hers.** *Another of my Fisher-Price analogies: imagine putting a Spanish-speaking person in a room with a German-speaking person. How successful would their efforts at communication be without one of them learning the other's language or mode of communicating?*

Early on, I was told by well-meaning people that I should only agree with her when it was "honest," and that I should gently redirect her when she was confused. I understand the intention behind that advice. But in practice, I've found that staying with her inside her reality is far less stressful for both of us — and it allows for more connection, not less.

When my mom is scared, I don't explain why she shouldn't be. I reassure her.

If she's worried that something isn't safe, I tell her it's been taken care of — the windows are locked, the doors are secure, everything is okay.

If she starts talking about moving a wall from one room to another, I don't argue the logistics. I say, "Sure — we'll tackle that tomorrow."

Tomorrow, in her world, is always a safe answer.

She isn't trying to be irrational. She's trying to make sense of a world that no longer behaves predictably. Asking her to converse in my reality only highlights what she's lost and almost always stops the communication process. Staying with her in hers preserves what's left.

When the Question Is About Someone Who Has Died

This comes up most painfully when a spouse or partner has passed away.

Your loved one may ask — repeatedly — where their husband or wife is. And you may feel compelled to explain, over and over, that they've died. I did that at first. I told my mom the truth in the beginning.

But over time, I realized something important:

She wasn't remembering that she asked.

She wasn't remembering the answer.

She was re-experiencing the loss.

Hour after hour. Day after day.

Now, when she asks where he is, I say he's out running errands.

Is that technically true? No.

Is it kind? In our case, yes.

I believe she knows, somewhere deep inside, that he's gone. But there is nothing to be gained — for her or for me — by reopening that wound again and again. Reminding her repeatedly doesn't help her grieve. It simply creates fresh pain without context or resolution.

This approach may not feel right for everyone. Family dynamics matter. Beliefs matter. What matters most is reducing suffering — not adhering to a rigid rulebook.

Connection Over Correction

Dementia changes how a person experiences reality. Communication isn't about accuracy anymore — it's about emotional safety.

When I meet my mom where she is:

- She feels calmer

- She engages more

- We have more moments of connection

She doesn't know how to converse in my world anymore.

So I step into hers — and we meet there.

Quick Communication Reset (When Everything Is Going Sideways)

When a conversation starts to escalate:

- Pause and lower your voice instead of raising your volume.

- Step closer if it feels safe, or give a bit more space if they seem cornered.

- Offer reassurance first ("You're safe. I'm here with you."), then any explanation.

- Change one thing: the topic, the room, the task, or your own body position.

☐ Ask yourself, "What might they be feeling right now?" more than "What are they saying?"

A Caregiver's Voice

I remember the day I realized that my mom could no longer order her meal at a restaurant. She looked at the menu, became instantly overwhelmed, and began to cry. I learned to order her favorite from the available selections. A good thing to remember is that our loved ones sometimes lose their ability to taste or discern exactly what they're eating. So just do your best.

Instead of:

"Do you remember what we talked about yesterday?"

Try:

"It's okay. We'll figure this out together."

Instead of:

"Do you want soup, a sandwich, or pasta?"

Try:

"I made soup. Let's have some together."

Offer Reassurance Before Information

Fear often comes before confusion. A calm tone and gentle reassurance can settle emotions even if words don't fully land.

When Emotions Run High

Agitation, anxiety, or argumentativeness often increase when a person feels rushed, misunderstood, or overwhelmed. When this happens, reasoning usually doesn't help.

What *does* help:

- Slowing down
- Lowering your voice
- Acknowledging feelings without agreeing with false beliefs
- Redirecting attention rather than confronting

For example:

"I can see you're upset. You're safe right now."

Validation doesn't mean agreeing with inaccuracies—it means acknowledging emotion.

When Your Loved One Argues or Becomes Defensive

Arguing is often a response to feeling threatened or misunderstood.

You might try:

- Letting go of facts and focusing on emotion
- Acknowledging feelings without agreeing or correcting (i.e., by saying, "Oh, really?" or "That must've been scary")
- Changing the environment or topic
- Stepping away briefly if tension escalates

You don't need to win the conversation. You need to reduce distress.

Repetition Isn't Defiance

One of the most exhausting parts of communication is repetition. The same question is asked dozens of times. The same worry resurfaces again and again.

This isn't stubbornness or intentional behavior. It's the brain losing the ability to store new information.

Responding with frustration often increases anxiety. Responding with reassurance—even if it feels repetitive—can prevent escalation.

Sometimes the *emotion* behind the question matters more than the answer.

When Conversations Stop Working, You Might Try This

When Your Loved One Repeats the Same Question

Repeated questions are rarely about memory alone. They're often about anxiety, confusion, or the need for reassurance. This is one of those lessons dementia teaches repeatedly — because repetition itself is part of the disease.

You might try:

- Answering calmly, even if it's the tenth time

- Writing the answer down where they can see it *(My mom quickly lost her ability to read early in her journey, so this didn't work for me.)*
- Redirecting gently rather than correcting
- Offering reassurance instead of information

Correcting rarely helps. Comfort often does.

Responding to Sundowning-Related Communication Changes

As discussed earlier, communication often becomes more difficult in the late afternoon or evening. During these times:

- Confusion increases
- Emotional regulation decreases
- Language may deteriorate

Expect less. Simplify more. Reduce stimulation. A gentle presence may be more effective than conversation.

This is not regression—it's fatigue.

Handling Suicidal Statements or Distressing Language

Some caregivers are shocked when a loved one expresses a desire to die or makes statements about wanting to disappear. These moments are frightening and emotionally heavy.

Such statements may reflect:

- Depression
- Fear
- Loss of control

- Confusion rather than intent

They should always be taken seriously—but not necessarily literally.

If statements are frequent, specific, or escalating, involve medical professionals immediately. If they are occasional expressions of distress, respond with reassurance and presence rather than panic.

You don't need to solve the feeling. You need to acknowledge it and seek support.

A Caregiver's Voice

I had to unlearn the instinct to explain and correct. This was a big one for me! The more I tried to explain so that things would make sense, the more distressed my loved one became. And, it's important to note that she didn't retain the new information in any case. Letting go of being right was painful—but it also brought more peace than I expected.

When Communication Stops Making Sense

As dementia progresses, words may lose meaning altogether. Communication may become fragmented, nonsensical, or largely nonverbal.

At that point, connection shifts again—to:

- Tone of voice
- Facial expression
- Touch (when welcomed)
- Familiar routines

Presence becomes the language.

Reflection Prompts

You don't need to answer every question. Use what feels helpful and leave the rest.

- When conversations go badly, what usually sets things off—my words, their fear, the timing, or something else?
- How do I feel when I stop correcting the facts and focus on comfort instead?
- What phrases or tones seem to calm my loved one, even a little?
- What phrases or habits of mine tend to make things worse, even when I don't mean to?
- How does it change things when I remember that difficult behaviors are often signs of unmet needs, not intentional hurt?
- Who could I practice new communication approaches with, so I don't feel so alone in learning this?

A Gentle Reminder

You are learning a new language in the middle of a crisis. No one does that perfectly.

There will be days when the best words still lead to tears or anger. That does not mean you failed. It means the disease is loud.

Every time you choose comfort over correction, you are protecting connection—even if the outcome isn't neat or peaceful.

You are allowed to try, adjust, and try again. That is what learning looks like here.

Looking Ahead

Communication is foundational. It shapes every other aspect of caregiving—from daily routines to medical decisions to emotional connection.

As the disease progresses, caregiving becomes more physical, more intimate, and more demanding. Tasks that once felt simple—bathing, dressing, toileting—can become sources of fear or resistance.

In the next chapter, we'll discuss the realities of daily care at home, including the challenges caregivers are often unprepared for—and how to address them with dignity, safety, and compassion.

Chapter 4 — Daily Caregiving Realities at Home

There often comes a point when caregiving shifts from *watching and supporting* to *doing*.

Daily life becomes more hands-on. Tasks that were once automatic—getting dressed, eating, bathing, using the bathroom—now require guidance, patience, or physical help. And with that shift comes a new layer of grief, exhaustion, and responsibility that many caregivers are unprepared for.

If this chapter feels heavy, it's because this stage is heavy.

If you haven't already, you may want to revisit the "Quick Home Safety Checklist" in Chapter 1. As dementia progresses, safety needs often change—and what once felt unnecessary may now offer peace of mind.

When Motivation Disappears

One of the most confusing changes caregivers notice is a loss of initiative. Your loved one may spend much of the day sleeping, sitting quietly, or showing little interest in activities they once enjoyed.

This isn't just laziness or depression. Dementia affects the brain's ability to initiate action. Even simple tasks can feel overwhelming when the steps can't be sequenced internally.

Encouragement helps—but pressure often doesn't. Gentle prompts, predictable routines, and lowering expectations can reduce frustration on both sides.

Some days, simply being awake and safe is enough.

When Your Loved One Resists Bathing: What May Help

Bathing resistance is one of the most common and distressing challenges caregivers face. It's also one of the most misunderstood.

What looks like stubbornness or refusal is often fear.

For someone with dementia, bathing can feel disorienting, threatening, or humiliating. Water may sound loud and overwhelming. Slippery surfaces can feel unsafe. Being undressed can trigger vulnerability or shame. Some people experience a genuine fear of drowning, even in shallow water.

If bathing becomes a struggle, you might try:

- **Changing the timing**
  Some people tolerate bathing better earlier in the day, when they're less fatigued or confused.

- **Simplifying the process**
  Explaining one step at a time — or not explaining at all — can reduce overwhelm.

- **Offering choices without pressure**
  "Would you like to wash your face or your hands first?" offers control without requiring complex decisions.

- **Preserving warmth and modesty**
  Warm the room. Use towels or robes to keep the body

covered as much as possible.

- **Rethinking what "counts" as a bath**
  Sponge baths, no-rinse cleansers, or washing on different days are valid alternatives.

- **Letting go of frequency**
  Fewer baths with less distress may be better than daily battles.

If bathing remains traumatic despite adjustments, it's okay to pause and reassess. Cleanliness matters — but emotional safety matters too. This is not a battle you have to win. You may want to keep adult cleansing wipes and an antibacterial ointment on hand. They'll come in handy.

And if resistance escalates or becomes unsafe, it may be a signal that additional help — or a different care environment — is needed.

That realization is not failure. It's information.

When Your Loved One Refuses to Eat

Loss of appetite can stem from confusion, depression, physical changes, or the brain's declining ability to interpret hunger.

You might try:

- Offering smaller, more frequent meals
- Serving familiar or favorite foods
- Reducing distractions during meals
- Letting go of "balanced" meals in favor of calories
- Eating together to model behavior

If eating becomes unsafe or stops altogether, this may signal
disease progression — not neglect.

When Clothing Changes Become a Battle

Refusing to change clothes often stems from comfort, routine, or
a sense of loss of control.

You might try:

- Buying duplicate favorite outfits
- Choosing soft, easy-to-remove clothing
- Offering limited choices
- Linking clothing changes to routine activities

This is often about familiarity, not defiance.

Incontinence: What's Normal and What to Expect

Incontinence is one of the most emotionally difficult changes for
caregivers to navigate. It can bring embarrassment, discomfort,
and a sense of loss of dignity—for both of you.

Yes, incontinence is common in dementia. It may appear
gradually or suddenly and often worsens as the disease
progresses.

This change is neurological, not behavioral. The brain loses the
ability to recognize signals or respond in a timely manner.

Planning ahead—protective bedding, clothing choices, bathroom
routines—can reduce stress. So you can let go of the idea that
this is something your loved one is doing *to* you.

It's something happening *to* them. Invest in mattress pads for wetting and adult diapers.

A Caregiver's Voice

I've read many times that people have a hard time emotionally with adult diapers. Just think of them as underwear. It's a critical need to help your loved one keep their dignity and reduce stress during clean-up.

When Incontinence Causes Distress

Incontinence is deeply tied to dignity.

You might try:

- Maintaining calm, neutral reactions
- Using absorbent products before accidents occur
- Watching for patterns
- Preserving privacy as much as possible

Shame increases distress. Calm reduces it.

When Sundowning Takes Over the Evenings

Late-day confusion and agitation are common.

You might try:

- Maintaining a predictable routine
- Increasing light in the late afternoon
- Reducing stimulation
- Offering calming activities
- Avoiding late-day naps if possible

Not every evening will be manageable. That's not a reflection of effort.

Developing and maintaining consistent routines is so much more valuable than I understood at first. In doing so, you may see fewer outbursts, more relaxation, and more participation. I had to learn the connection between the routine and positive outcomes the hard way.

When Injuries Happen at Home

Falls and injuries are frightening, and they happen more often than caregivers expect—even in familiar environments.

If a fall occurs:

- Stay calm
- Assess for injury
- Seek medical attention when needed
- Document what happened

Falls are not failures. They are part of the risk landscape of dementia.

Preventive steps—lighting, clear pathways, mobility aids—can help, but they can't eliminate all risk. Try to release self-blame when accidents occur.

Keeping the Home Safe: Reducing Risk Without Turning It Into a Facility

As dementia progresses, the home environment can quietly become more dangerous — not because anyone is careless, but because the brain is changing how it interprets space, depth, judgment, and risk.

Caregivers often struggle with this section of the journey because safety changes feel symbolic. Adding locks, removing rugs, or changing routines can feel like crossing an emotional line — as if acknowledging safety needs means acknowledging decline.

But home safety isn't about giving up independence.

It's about **reducing unnecessary risk** so daily life can continue with less fear, fewer emergencies, and more stability.

You don't need to do everything at once. And you don't need to make your home look medical or institutional. Small, thoughtful changes can make a meaningful difference.

Why Safety Needs Change

Dementia affects:

- Balance and coordination
- Depth perception and visual processing
- Judgment and impulse control
- The ability to recognize danger

A stove, a staircase, a bathroom, or a doorway that once felt familiar may now be confusing or threatening — or falsely safe.

Most injuries at home happen not during dramatic events, but during **ordinary moments**:

- Standing up too quickly
- Reaching for something familiar
- Walking to the bathroom at night
- Trying to "help" with tasks they once handled easily

Planning ahead reduces the chance that a small moment becomes a crisis.

Home Safety Is an Ongoing Process

Safety is not a one-time checklist. It changes as abilities change.

What felt unnecessary six months ago may now offer peace of mind. Revisiting safety doesn't mean things are "getting worse." It means you're responding to reality with care.

Quick Guide: Home Safety for Dementia Caregivers

(Reduce risk, preserve dignity, protect both of you)

General Living Areas

- Remove loose rugs, cords, or clutter that could cause falls
- Improve lighting, especially in hallways and corners
- Use nightlights in bedrooms, bathrooms, and walkways
- Secure heavy furniture and televisions to prevent tipping

Bathroom Safety

- Install grab bars near toilets and in showers

- Use non-slip mats in tubs and on bathroom floors
- Consider a shower chair or handheld showerhead
- Adjust water heater temperature to prevent burns

Kitchen Safety

- Store sharp objects, cleaning supplies, and medications out of sight
- Consider stove safety knobs, automatic shut-offs, or supervised cooking only
- Unplug appliances when not in use, if confusion increases
- Monitor for forgotten food, overheating, or unsafe combinations

Bedroom Safety

- Ensure the bed is at a safe height for standing
- Remove clutter between the bed and bathroom
- Consider motion-sensor lights for nighttime movement
- Use simple bedding to reduce confusion

Stairs & Entryways

- Install handrails on both sides of stairs
- Mark step edges with contrasting tape if depth perception is impaired
- Secure doors discreetly if wandering becomes a concern
- Use door alarms or chimes if needed — not to restrict, but to alert

Medication Safety

- Use a pill organizer filled by one designated person
- Store medications out of sight and reach

- Keep an up-to-date medication list for emergencies and appointments

Emergency Preparedness

- Keep emergency numbers visible for caregivers
- Have a plan for falls or sudden illness
- Consider medical alert systems if appropriate
- Keep identification accessible in case of wandering

A Gentle Perspective on Safety Changes

Every safety adjustment comes with emotion — for caregivers and for the person receiving care. Resistance doesn't always mean disagreement; sometimes it means fear, loss, or confusion.

If a safety change causes distress:

- Pause and reassess
- Introduce it gradually
- Reframe it as convenience or comfort rather than necessity

You are not taking something away.

You are making space for continued living.

When Home Safety Is No Longer Enough

There may come a point when safety risks outweigh what can reasonably be managed at home — even with modifications and support.

Recognizing that moment is not failure.

It is information.

This is often when caregivers begin considering additional help, in-home care, or alternative living environments — a decision we'll explore more deeply in later chapters.

For now, know this: **every step you take to make the home safer is an act of love**, even when it's emotionally hard.

When Wandering or Exit-Seeking Appears

Wandering often reflects restlessness, anxiety, or unmet needs.

You might try:

- Securing doors discreetly
- Providing safe pacing areas
- Redirecting with purpose ("Can you help me with…")
- Ensuring identification is worn

Wandering is a safety issue, not a behavior issue.

When Sleep Patterns Reverse

Day-night confusion can exhaust caregivers.

You might try:

- Increasing daytime activity
- Limiting or eliminating caffeine
- Maintaining consistent sleep routines
- Discussing sleep concerns with providers

Chronic sleep deprivation for caregivers is not sustainable — help is warranted.

Quick Guide: Daily Care Log (To Notice Patterns, Not Perfection)

Use this as a simple snapshot, not a report card.

Morning

- Approximate wake-up time:
- Medications taken (yes / no / issues):
- Mood and alertness (calm, anxious, agitated, sleepy):
- Any falls, confusion, or concerning behaviors:

Midday

- Meals or snacks eaten (what went well, what didn't):
- Activities (even small ones: TV, short walk, sitting outside):
- Rest or naps (how long, how they woke up):

Evening / Night

- Sundowning signs (pacing, fear, agitation, asking to "go home"):
- Strategies that helped (lighting, music, routine, reassurance):
- Sleep start time and number of nighttime awakenings:

☐   1–2 behaviors or changes I want to bring up next time:

☐   One thing that felt especially hard today:

☐   One thing that went better than expected:

Behavioral Changes That Feel Unmanageable

Some behaviors cross into territory caregivers never imagined they would face: breaking objects, unsafe actions, inappropriate behaviors, or fecal smearing.

These behaviors are not intentional, malicious, or personal. They are symptoms of brain changes affecting impulse control, sensory processing, and awareness.

What looks like indifference or disengagement is often apathy— a neurological symptom, not a choice.

Responding with punishment or logic rarely helps. Safety, supervision, and professional guidance matter more than discipline.

If behaviors become overwhelming or dangerous, it's okay to say: *This is more than I can manage alone.*

Physical Changes Caregivers Will See

As dementia progresses, caregivers may notice:

- Changes in gait or balance
- Weight loss or changes in appetite
- Difficulty swallowing

- Increased sleep
- Reduced mobility

These changes can be gradual or sudden. They are often distressing because they signal progression—but they are not reflections of caregiving quality.

Your role isn't to stop progression. It's to respond with care.

Caring for Yourself While Caring for Them

Daily caregiving takes a toll. Many caregivers develop physical symptoms: back pain, fatigue, insomnia, headaches, and anxiety. These are not signs of weakness—they are signs of sustained stress.

Ignoring your own needs doesn't make you stronger. It makes burnout more likely.

Support—whether through respite care, in-home help, or simply asking someone to sit with your loved one—protects *both* of you.

For more information on caregiver burnout, see Chapter 6 (family dynamics) and Appendix B resources.

A Caregiver's Voice

There were days when getting through basic tasks felt like an impossible mountain. I learned that lowering expectations didn't mean giving up—it meant choosing peace where I could.

Reflection Prompts

You don't need to answer these at once. Choose what feels most relevant today.

- Which daily tasks drain me the most right now, physically or emotionally?
- Where am I pushing myself past my limits out of guilt or fear?
- What small changes (timing, tools, asking for help) might make one hard task a little easier?
- When something goes wrong—a fall, resistance, an outburst—how do I talk to myself about it?
- What would it sound like to speak to myself with the same compassion I offer my loved ones?
- What signs tell me I'm nearing burnout, and what support could I reach for sooner, not later?

A Gentle Reminder

Your body is part of this story too. Exhaustion, pain, and overwhelm are not character flaws—they are signals.

There is no prize for doing every task alone or for pretending this is easy.

Choosing easier methods, accepting help, or changing routines is not "giving up." It is protecting both of you.

You are allowed to make care sustainable, not heroic.

Looking Ahead

Daily care often stretches caregivers to their limits. Over time, many begin to wonder whether home is still the safest or most sustainable option.

That question doesn't mean you've failed. It means you're paying attention.

In the next chapter, we'll talk about the emotional cost of caregiving—the guilt, grief, fear, and isolation that so often go unspoken—and why tending to your emotional health matters just as much as tending to theirs.

A Final Permission

You are allowed to experiment. Remember my Fisher-Price analogy about taste buds. Not every solution will work for every patient.

You are allowed to stop what isn't working.

You are allowed to ask for help before you collapse.

There is no perfect way to care for someone with dementia. There is only what works for your loved one and is *enough* for now.

Chapter 5 — The Caregiver's Emotional World

If you came to this section because you started in the "If You're in Crisis" page at the front of the book, I'm glad you're here.

There is a kind of grief that doesn't wait for death.

It arrives early, lingers quietly, and settles into daily life. It shows up while you're still caregiving, still showing up, still doing everything you can—yet already mourning what's slipping away.

This is dementia grief, and it is ongoing.

Grieving Someone Who Is Still Alive

One of the most confusing and painful aspects of dementia caregiving is grieving while the person you love is still here. Their body remains. Their presence remains. But pieces of who they were—their humor, insight, memory, or emotional availability—begin to fade.

You don't just grieve once. You grieve in layers over the timespan of the dementia journey.

You grieve:

- The loss of shared memories
- The loss of future plans
- The loss of conversation and recognition
- The loss of ease and familiarity

This grief often goes unrecognized by others, which can make it feel even heavier. People may say, "At least they're still alive," without understanding that what you're grieving is not a single event—it's a continuous, daily process.

Guilt: The Companion Nobody Talks About

- Guilt threads itself through nearly every aspect of caregiving.
- Guilt for feeling impatient.
- Guilt for wishing for rest.
- Guilt for wanting your life back.
- Guilt for considering help—or placement.
- Guilt for feeling resentful, angry, or numb.

These feelings don't mean you love your loved one less. They mean you are human, stretched beyond what most people ever have to face.

Guilt often grows in silence. Naming it reduces its power.

When Heartbreak Becomes Overwhelming

There is a level of heartbreak in dementia caregiving that goes beyond sadness.

It's the kind that takes your breath away. The kind that settles into your chest and makes it hard to move forward, even when you know you must. The kind that leaves you staring at the ceiling at night, wondering how much more you can carry.

This heartbreak is not dramatic. It is quiet, relentless, and cumulative.

Grief in dementia is ongoing, but it's also layered with fear—fear of what's coming next, fear of making the wrong decision, fear of losing yourself along the way. Over time, that fear can harden into anger or collapse into numbness. Guilt weaves through it all, convincing you that any moment of relief, resentment, or desire for escape makes you a bad person.

This emotional weight can feel paralyzing.

Some caregivers describe feeling stuck—unable to imagine the future, unable to fully live in the present, and unable to step away. Others feel constantly on edge, emotionally raw, or dangerously depleted. These aren't personal failures. They are warning signs of a system under too much strain.

The Collision of Grief, Fear, Anger, and Guilt

These emotions don't appear neatly or separately. They collide.

- **Grief** mourns what's already gone and what will never be.
- **Fear** scans constantly for the next loss or crisis.
- **Anger** pushes back against the unfairness of it all.
- **Guilt** questions every thought, feeling, and decision.

Together, they can trap caregivers in a cycle of self-judgment and emotional isolation. You may find yourself asking:

- *Why can't I handle this better?*
- *What kind of person thinks these things?*
- *How am I supposed to keep going?*

If you've had moments where the pain feels unbearable—or where you've wondered whether you can survive this journey—you are not alone. And you are not weak.

When You're at the End of Your Rope

There is a point where heartbreak stops being something you "manage" and becomes something you need help carrying.

If you feel emotionally numb, constantly overwhelmed, or trapped in despair, it's important to know this: **needing help does not mean you've failed**. It means you are human, responding to prolonged trauma.

Support might look like:

- Talking with a therapist or counselor familiar with caregiver stress. *(I always tell people to interview a therapist the way you would for a job. Ask if they've worked with dementia and caregiver stress before. You don't need a full appointment to ask initial questions — a phone message is enough. If they don't return your call in a reasonable time, that may be an indication of their responsiveness. If it's not the right fit, you are allowed to find another.)*
- Joining a caregiver support group, in person or online (I am building an online community at www.dementiacarejourney.com for those who don't want to be overwhelmed by social media.)
- Telling a trusted person, honestly, how bad it feels
- Asking for respite—even if it feels impossible

If at any point you feel unsafe, hopeless, or afraid of what you might do, that is not something to push through alone. Reaching out for immediate support is an act of courage, not weakness.

Five-Minute Emotional Check-In (For You)

Use this when everything feels like too much, or once a day if you can.

- Name it: "Right now I feel…" (angry, numb, terrified, hopeless, overwhelmed, blank).
- Locate it: Where do I feel this in my body? (chest, jaw, stomach, head, shoulders).
- Rate it: On a scale of 1–10, how intense is it right now?
- Soften it: What is one small thing I can do in the next 10 minutes to soften this a little? (step outside, drink water, text someone, cry in peace, sit in silence).
- Tell someone: Who could know how bad this feels—without fixing it, just witnessing it?

Making Space for the Pain Without Letting It Consume You

You don't need to make the heartbreak meaningful. You don't need to grow from it. You don't need to be grateful for the lessons it teaches.

What you need is permission to acknowledge how devastating this can be—and to protect yourself within it.

Caring for someone with dementia is not just emotionally difficult. It can be **traumatizing**. Naming that truth matters.

Fear and Hypervigilance

Many caregivers live in a constant state of alertness.

You worry about falls, wandering, medical emergencies, agitation, and what might happen when you're not there. Even when things are calm, your body may stay tense—braced for the next crisis.

This kind of chronic vigilance takes a toll. Anxiety, sleep disturbances, irritability, and difficulty relaxing are common. Over time, your nervous system can forget what "off duty" feels like.

This isn't a weakness. It's biology responding to prolonged stress.

Anger, Resentment, and Shame

Anger is one of the most stigmatized emotions in caregiving—and one of the most common. Some caregivers feel anger toward the person with dementia themselves—especially when behaviors feel unfair or relentless—and then feel deep shame for it. This, too, is common, and it does not cancel love.

You may feel angry at:

- The disease
- The situation
- Other family members
- The healthcare system
- Your loved one
- Yourself

Anger often masks deeper emotions: grief, fear, helplessness, and exhaustion. When anger is judged instead of understood, shame often follows.

Shame thrives in isolation. Compassion interrupts it.

The Loneliness of Being "The One"

Caregiving can be profoundly isolating.

Even when surrounded by people, you may feel unseen or misunderstood. Friends may pull away. Family members may disagree, disengage, or minimize what you're experiencing. Conversations drift toward normal life while yours feels suspended.

This isolation isn't always intentional—but it is deeply felt.

You may begin to feel like no one truly understands what your days look like, what you're carrying, or how heavy the responsibility feels.

When Caregiving Affects the Body

Emotional stress doesn't stay emotional. It shows up physically.

Many caregivers experience:

- Chronic fatigue
- Headaches or muscle pain
- Gastrointestinal issues
- Sleep disruption
- Weakened immune response

Your body is not betraying you. It's signaling that the load is heavy.

Listening to these signals is an act of care, not indulgence.

Meaning in the Middle of Loss

One of the hardest questions caregivers wrestle with is: *How do I make sense of this?*

Meaning doesn't come from pretending this journey is noble or redemptive. It comes from presence. From showing up. From advocating when your loved one cannot. From choosing compassion—even when it hurts.

Meaning is not something you find. It's what you give to the experience.

A Caregiver's Voice

There are moments when I'm afraid and worry that I'm not doing the right thing for my Mom. Am I doing enough? Am I making the right decision? There were other moments when I felt ashamed of how tired, angry, or resentful I was. It took time to understand that these feelings weren't a reflection of my love—they were a reflection of how much I was carrying.

Reflection Prompts

These questions are not meant to be answered all at once. Some may feel heavy. Go slowly. Stop when you need to.

- What emotions show up most often for me in caregiving—grief, fear, anger, numbness, something else?
- Which feelings do I allow myself to show, and which ones do I quickly hide or judge?
- In what moments do I feel most alone in this, and what (or who) helps that loneliness soften even a little?

- How do I talk to myself after I lose my patience or feel resentful—do I punish myself, or can I offer even a little compassion?
- What are my personal warning signs that I am nearing the end of my rope?
- What kinds of support (professional, spiritual, practical, social) feel most accessible to me right now—and which feel out of reach but still worth exploring?

If You're Feeling Overwhelmed or Unsafe

If you are feeling hopeless, emotionally numb, or afraid of what you might do, **please reach out for immediate support**. You do not have to carry this alone.

- **U.S. Suicide & Crisis Lifeline:** Call or text **988** (24/7)
- If you are outside the U.S., local crisis hotlines can be found through your country's health services
- For dementia-specific caregiver support, education, and helplines, contact the **Alzheimer's Association** (www.alz.org)

Reaching out is not a failure. It is a response to pain that deserves care.

A Gentle Reminder

The way you are feeling is not a character flaw. It is a human response to prolonged stress, loss, and responsibility.

Grief, anger, fear, and even wishing this were over do not make you a bad caregiver. They make you honest.

Needing help—professional, practical, spiritual, or emergency—is not proof that you've failed. It is proof that you have been carrying more than one person's share for a very long time.

You are allowed to be cared for, too.

Looking Ahead

Caregiving doesn't happen in isolation. Families are systems, and dementia has a way of exposing old dynamics and creating new tensions.

In the next chapter, we'll explore family relationships, sibling dynamics, advocacy, and why people often respond so differently to the same diagnosis—and how to protect yourself while navigating it.

Chapter 6 — Family Dynamics and Advocacy

Dementia doesn't just affect one person—it reverberates through families. Old roles resurface. Longstanding tensions reappear. Differences in values, proximity, denial, and coping styles become painfully visible.

Many caregivers are unprepared for how difficult this part of the journey can be.

Why Families React So Differently

One of the most confusing aspects of dementia caregiving is watching people you love respond in ways that feel unhelpful—or even hurtful.

Some family members:

- Minimize symptoms or deny there's a problem
- Avoid involvement entirely
- Criticize decisions without offering help
- Disagree about care, money, or placement
- Appear detached or overly optimistic

These reactions are rarely about you. They're about their own relationship with your loved one. They're about how each person copes with fear, grief, guilt, and a sense of loss of control.

Keep in mind that family members each have a different set of "taste buds" and have had their own and varied experiences with your loved one. There is an emotional history that feeds into who they became as adults. People protect themselves in different ways. Some step forward. Others step back. Neither response is a reliable measure of love.

When You Become "The One"

In many families, one person gradually becomes *the caregiver*—even if no one ever officially agrees to it.

If that's you, you may find yourself:

- Coordinating appointments
- Managing medications
- Handling finances or paperwork
- Making safety decisions
- Absorbing emotional fallout

Being "the one" can feel isolating and overwhelming, especially when others second-guess decisions without sharing the workload.

You are allowed to acknowledge how heavy this role is.

Setting Boundaries Without Burning Bridges

Boundaries are not punishments. They are protections.

You may need to set limits around:

- How much input others have
- How criticism is handled
- What decisions are non-negotiable
- How often do you explain or justify choices

Boundaries don't require everyone's agreement to be valid. They require clarity and consistency.

You don't have to convince everyone—you have to keep your loved one safe and yourself functional.

Conversation Starters for Hard Family Talks

Use these as templates; tweak them to fit your family's language.

- "I can't safely do this alone anymore. We need to either share the load differently or rethink the plan."
- "This is what the doctor is recommending. Can we talk about how to support that, even if we feel differently about it?"
- "I'm not asking you to agree with every decision. I'm asking you to help me make sure Mom/Dad is safe and cared for."
- "When you say 'let me know if you need anything,' I'm not always sure what to ask for. Here are two things that would actually help..."
- "It's hard for me when I feel second-guessed but not supported. How can we share concerns in a way that still feels like we're on the same team?"

Advocating for Your Loved One

As dementia progresses, caregivers often become translators, defenders, and decision-makers.

Advocacy may include:

- Speaking up during medical appointments
- Ensuring concerns are taken seriously

- Clarifying symptoms and behaviors
- Pushing for reassessment when things change
- Coordinating between providers

This can feel intimidating—especially when you're exhausted or unfamiliar with the system. Remember: no one knows your loved one better than you do.

Advocacy isn't about being difficult. It's about being accurate.

Navigating Human and Social Services

Many caregivers don't realize how many resources exist—or how hard they can be to access without guidance.

Helpful starting points often include:

- Your county's senior services or human services department
- Local aging or disability resource centers
- Caregiver support programs
- Legal or financial counseling referrals

For education, support groups, and a caregiver helpline, the **Alzheimer's Association** is a widely used resource. Even if your loved one doesn't have Alzheimer's specifically, their materials and support services are often applicable across dementias.

Asking for help navigating these systems is not a weakness—it's a skill.

Documentation Is Critical

When families disagree or systems become complex, documentation protects everyone.

Keep records of:

- Medical visits and recommendations
- Behavioral changes or incidents
- Medication changes and responses
- Safety concerns
- Financial or legal decisions

Documentation creates continuity, reduces confusion, and supports advocacy when memories—or opinions—differ.

Protecting Yourself Emotionally

Family conflict can drain caregivers faster than physical tasks.

You are allowed to:

- Step away from arguments
- Decline conversations that go nowhere
- Seek outside validation and support
- Choose peace over consensus

You don't have to carry everyone else's feelings on top of your own.

A Caregiver's Voice

I learned that not everyone would walk this road with me—and that hurt more than I expected. Letting go of the need for agreement didn't mean letting go of the relationship. It meant choosing what my loved one needed most.

Reflection Prompts

You don't need to answer these at once. Choose what feels most relevant right now.

- What role have I taken on in my family around caregiving—organizer, doer, peacemaker, scapegoat, something else?
- Where do I feel most supported by family, and where do I feel most alone or undermined?
- What boundaries do I wish I could set—and what fears come up when I imagine actually setting them?
- How do old family patterns (who decides, who avoids, who fixes) show up in our current caregiving decisions?
- What kind of help do I truly need (time, money, presence, advocacy), and who might realistically be able to offer each piece?
- If someone I loved were in my position, what would I want their family to do differently?

A Gentle Reminder

You are navigating your loved one's illness and your family's history at the same time. No one is perfectly equipped for that.

Other people's denial, distance, or criticism are about their own limits and fears, not your worth or effort.

You are allowed to set boundaries, ask directly for what you need, and step back from arguments that go nowhere. Protecting your energy is part of protecting your loved one.

Looking Ahead

As caregiving continues, questions about finances, insurance, and long-term planning often move from "someday" to *now*. These conversations can feel overwhelming—but understanding options early can prevent crisis decisions later.

In the next chapter, we'll talk about financial planning, insurance, and resources—what to know, what to ask, and why timing matters.

Chapter 7 — Financial Planning and Legal Protection

There is a moment in most caregiving journeys when "we'll deal with that later" quietly becomes *now*.

It may be triggered by a missed bill, a medical emergency, a disagreement with a provider, or the realization that decisions are being made without clear authority. Financial and legal planning often feels intimidating—not because caregivers don't care, but because the stakes feel so high.

This chapter isn't about mastering the system. It's about protecting your loved one, protecting yourself, and preventing avoidable crises.

Why Financial and Legal Planning Matters Early

Dementia is progressive, but decision-making ability often declines unevenly. Someone may seem capable in conversation while quietly losing the ability to manage finances, understand contracts, or make informed medical choices.

Planning early:

- Preserves your loved one's autonomy
- Reduces family conflict later
- Prevents court involvement when possible
- Gives caregivers authority to act when it's needed most

Waiting doesn't keep things the same. It often narrows options.

Understanding the Financial Landscape of Care

Caregiving is expensive—financially, emotionally, and physically.

Common costs include:

- In-home care (especially round-the-clock care)
- Medical co-pays and prescriptions
- Home modifications
- Transportation
- Memory care or skilled nursing facilities

Round-the-clock in-home care can quickly exceed the cost of residential care, yet families often choose it because it feels less disruptive. There is no universally "right" choice—only what works for your situation, values, and resources.

Knowing the numbers early allows for informed decisions rather than emergency ones.

Long-Term Care Insurance

If your loved one has long-term care insurance, review the policy as early as possible. If you don't already have a policy, it may be worth looking into as early as possible.

Important questions to ask:

- What types of care are covered?
- When does coverage begin?
- Is there an elimination period?
- What documentation is required?

These policies can be complex, and benefits are often delayed by paperwork. The average waiting period, or qualification period, for insurance coverage under long-term care policies is 90 days, meaning financial assistance is 3 months away. Starting early reduces frustration later.

Financial Resources and Assistance

Depending on location and eligibility, families may have access to:

- County or state senior services
- Medicaid or other assistance programs
- Veteran benefits
- Sliding-scale or subsidized services

Navigating these systems takes time and persistence. Asking for help navigating them is not a failure—it's often necessary.

Legal Planning: Documents That Protect Everyone

Legal documents are not about taking control away from your loved one. They are about ensuring their wishes are honored and their needs met when they can no longer speak or act for themselves.

These documents are most effective when completed **early**, while the person still has legal capacity.

Power of Attorney (Financial)

A financial power of attorney allows a designated person to:

- Pay bills
- Manage accounts

- Handle property or investments
- Sign legal or financial documents

Without this authority, caregivers may be unable to manage even basic financial tasks—even when everyone agrees it's necessary. Be sure that you or the identified person has signature authority over your loved one's bank accounts.

Healthcare Power of Attorney

A healthcare power of attorney designates someone to:

- Make medical decisions
- Communicate with providers
- Access medical information

This document becomes critical during emergencies or when your loved one can no longer understand or communicate medical choices.

Advance Directives / Living Wills

Advance directives outline preferences for medical care, particularly at the end of life.

They can address:

- Life-sustaining treatments
- Comfort-focused care
- Wishes around hospitalization

These documents don't eliminate grief—but they can reduce guilt and uncertainty when difficult decisions arise.

HIPAA Authorization

HIPAA laws protect patient privacy, but they can also unintentionally block caregivers from accessing information.

A HIPAA authorization allows healthcare providers to share information with designated individuals. Without it, even close family members may be excluded from conversations.

Guardianship or Conservatorship

When no legal authority exists—and a person can no longer make safe decisions—a court may appoint a guardian or conservator. In the U.S., the Social Security Administration requires guardianship authorization before discussing your loved one's situation.

This process:

- Can be expensive and time-consuming
- Often involves court oversight
- Is typically a last resort

Families sometimes pursue guardianship not because they failed to plan, but because planning wasn't possible earlier. It is a protective measure—not a moral judgment.

Guardianship: When a Power of Attorney Isn't Enough

Many families assume that once a Power of Attorney (POA) is in place, they can manage all aspects of their loved one's affairs. In most cases, that's true. However, there are situations where institutions may require more.

For example, the Social Security Administration does not recognize a Power of Attorney. Instead, they require you to apply to become a **Representative Payee** in order to manage your loved one's Social Security benefits. This is a separate process and may involve documentation and approval directly through the Social Security office.

In more complex situations — especially if legal documents were not completed early in the disease process — families may need to pursue **legal guardianship** (sometimes called conservatorship, depending on your state). Guardianship is a court-ordered arrangement granting someone the legal authority to make financial and/or medical decisions for a person who is no longer deemed capable of doing so.

Guardianship can be:

- Time-consuming
- Emotionally difficult
- Potentially expensive
- Public (since it involves court proceedings)

Because of this, it is typically considered a last resort when other planning tools — such as durable power of attorney, healthcare surrogate designation, and living wills — are not in place or are being challenged.

If dementia has already progressed to the point where your loved one can no longer legally sign documents, guardianship may be the only option available to ensure their safety and proper management of their affairs.

If you have legal documents in place, do you understand which institutions will honor them — and which will not?

Quick Guide: When to Consult an Elder Law Attorney

Consider speaking with an elder law attorney if:

- Your loved one did not complete POA or healthcare directives early.
- Family members disagree about decision-making.
- Financial exploitation is a concern.
- You're being told "We can't accept this POA."
- You are unsure whether guardianship may be necessary.

When Legal Planning Brings Up Family Conflict

Legal and financial decisions can surface deep family tensions.

Some relatives may:

- Disagree with decisions
- Feel excluded
- Question motives
- Resist acknowledging decline

Without these documents in place, your loved one is more susceptible to manipulation in line with someone else's agenda. Clear documentation protects not just finances, but relationships. It removes ambiguity and reduces the burden on caregivers to justify every decision.

A Caregiver's Voice

I didn't realize how quickly "we'll do this later" became "we can't do it at all now." Having the paperwork in place didn't make the situation easier—but it made it survivable.

Taking This One Step at a Time

You don't need to complete everything at once. Start with what feels most urgent. Ask professionals to explain things in plain language. Take breaks when it becomes too much.

Planning is not pessimism. It's care.

Quick Guide: If You Can Only Do a Few Things Right Now

You do not have to do everything at once. If you're overwhelmed, start small.

Choose one professional to contact:

- Elder law attorney, social worker, financial planner, or trusted advisor.

Gather basics before that call:

- Current list of medications, diagnosis (if known), income sources, major assets, and any existing legal documents.

Prioritize one document to address first:

- ☐ Often, a financial Power of Attorney or Healthcare Power of Attorney.

Ask three questions in any meeting:

- "What is most urgent?"
- "What can wait?"
- "What support exists to help us with this?"

Reflection Prompts

You don't need to answer everything here. Some of these questions may feel uncomfortable—and that's okay.

Facing the Reality of Planning

- ☐ What thoughts or emotions come up when I think about finances or legal planning?

- ☐ Have I been avoiding certain conversations because they feel overwhelming or scary?

- ☐ What feels most urgent right now—and what could wait?

Protecting, Not Controlling

- ☐ How do I feel about making decisions on behalf of my loved one?

- ☐ What fears come up around "taking away independence"?

- ☐ In what ways might planning actually protect my loved one's dignity and wishes?

Financial Stress and Limitations

- ☐ What financial concerns weigh most heavily on me?
- ☐ Am I comparing my situation to others in ways that increase guilt or shame?
- ☐ What resources might be available that I haven't explored yet?

Legal Readiness

- ☐ Which legal documents are already in place—and which are missing?
- ☐ What support would help me take the next step (an attorney, social worker, trusted advisor)?
- ☐ What would it feel like to have clearer authority during a crisis?

Giving Yourself Permission

- ☐ Am I holding myself to an unrealistic standard of preparedness?
- ☐ What would it look like to take this one step at a time?
- ☐ How can I see planning as an act of care rather than fear?

A Gentle Reminder

Planning for the future is not inviting disaster. It is putting cushions in place around a reality that is already hard.

Legal and financial documents do not measure how much you love someone. They simply give you the authority and protection to act on that love when things get complicated.

You are not responsible for predicting every possibility. You are only responsible for taking the next wise step with the information, energy, and resources you have today.

Looking Ahead

As care needs grow and resources stretch, many families begin to consider whether care at home is still sustainable—or safe.

In the next chapter, we'll talk about researching memory care and skilled facilities, what to ask, what to expect, and how to navigate one of the hardest decisions caregivers face.

Chapter 8 — Considering In-Home Caregivers, Memory Care, or Skilled Facilities

For many caregivers, the thought of placing a loved one in a facility brings immediate guilt and overwhelming sadness. Your loved one has said repeatedly that they don't ever want to be placed in a facility.

It can feel like a line you're not allowed to cross. A promise you didn't know you made but now feel bound to keep. Somewhere along the way, many caregivers absorb the belief that loving someone means caring for them yourself—no matter the cost.

That belief is powerful. And sometimes, it can be wrong.

If You're in Crisis About Placement, Start Here

If you're reading this because things feel unsafe at home right now, you don't need to read this entire chapter before taking action.

Start with:

- "When Home Is No Longer the Safest Place" (signs that safety is at risk).

- "A Decision Checklist: Is It Time to Consider a Facility?" (you don't have to check every box).

- "What to Expect Emotionally When You Consider Placement" (why guilt and relief often collide).

If one or more safety signs are happening now—frequent falls, wandering, medical crises you can't manage—it's okay to explore facilities before you feel "ready." Safety is not betrayal. It's care.

And sometimes the decision isn't driven by a single dramatic event, but by a quiet knowing that what worked before isn't working now. Whether this feels urgent or gradual, you may find yourself standing at a crossroads. Let's examine the options, benefits, cost implications, and any hurdles to help you make a choice that works best for you.

Why Care Decisions Change Over Time

Dementia is progressive, but not linear. What worked six months ago may not work now. Safety, dignity, and caregiver sustainability all matter—and choosing differently later is adaptation, not failure.

The Myth That You "Have" to Do This Yourself

Many caregivers feel an unspoken pressure to prove their love through endurance. To keep going no matter how exhausted, injured, or overwhelmed they become.

But dementia care is not just emotional—it's physical, medical, and constant.

Most family caregivers:

- Are not trained in safe transfers or lifting
- Are not equipped to manage medical emergencies alone
- Cannot provide 24/7 supervision indefinitely
- Are at real risk of injury themselves

Falls, infections, wandering, and agitation don't just endanger the person with dementia—they endanger the caregiver too. An injury that might have been minor in a supervised facility can become catastrophic at home.

Acknowledging this reality is not a failure. It's clarity.

Myths vs. Realities of Caregiving at Home

Myth: If I love them enough, I should be able to do this myself.

Reality: Love does not replace training, staffing, or medical support.

Myth: Placing them means I'm giving up.

Reality: Placement often means *changing* how you care, not stopping.

Myth: A facility will never care as family does.

Reality: Facilities provide structure, supervision, and expertise that families often can't sustain alone.

Myth: I should wait until I absolutely can't handle it anymore.

Reality: Waiting until a crisis often limits options and increases trauma for everyone.

Myth: Good caregivers sacrifice everything.

Reality: Sustainable care requires honesty about your limits. Your capacity is shaped by your health, your support system, your finances, and the history of your relationship. Sacrificing everything may feel noble in the moment, but over time, it

erodes stability, increases burnout, and can damage both of you.
Caring well does not require destroying yourself in the process.

The Reality of Relying on Family as Caregivers

Why This Is So Hard — Even with Love

- No formal training or crisis preparation
- High risk of falls and accidents
- Emotional decision-making under stress

The Hidden Costs

- Burnout
- Strained relationships
- Chronic guilt when something goes wrong

A Gentle Truth

- Love does not equal capacity
- Needing help is awareness, not failure

Reframing the Decision

- Care choices are about **supporting everyone involved**
- Safety and dignity apply to caregivers, too
- Changing course is part of responsible care

Considering In-Home Care Agencies

For many families, the first step away from doing everything
yourself is bringing help into the home. In-home care allows your
loved one to remain in familiar surroundings while receiving

support tailored to their needs—and, just as importantly, to yours.

This isn't a failure. It's recognizing that dementia care eventually exceeds what one person can sustainably manage alone.

What In-Home Care Actually Means

In-home care agencies provide trained caregivers who come to the home for scheduled blocks of time. Services can range from companionship and supervision to hands-on personal care.

Depending on the agency and the caregiver's credentials, support may include:

- Bathing, dressing, and grooming
- Toileting and incontinence care
- Meal preparation and feeding assistance
- Medication reminders
- Mobility assistance and transfers
- Light housekeeping
- Transportation to appointments
- Companionship and supervision
- Respite care so family caregivers can rest

Some agencies also provide licensed nurses for more medically complex needs, though that typically comes at a higher cost.

One of the greatest advantages of in-home care is flexibility. Services can often be scheduled:

- A few hours a week
- Several hours a day
- Overnight
- Around known stress points (like evenings or bath time)

You can increase or decrease hours as needs change. That ability to "program" care around your life — not the other way around — is often what makes this option appealing.

What It Typically Costs

Costs vary widely by region, but across the United States, in-home care typically ranges from: **$25–$35 per hour**

If care is needed:

- 20 hours per week → approximately $2,000–$3,000 per month
- 40 hours per week → approximately $4,000–$6,000 per month
- Around-the-clock care → $12,000+ per month

  ### A Caregiver's Voice

  When I first became responsible for my mom's care, I needed round-the-clock care for many reasons. The goal was getting her into a memory care facility, but I knew I had work to do before that could happen (i.e., checking coverage, visiting facilities, and the like). In-home care in our area ranged from $16,000 to $22,000/month. Not something we could do long-term. Neither my mother nor I could afford this, so we went through our savings quickly.

Costs rise quickly as supervision needs increase.

Long-term care insurance may cover a portion of in-home services, depending on the policy. Medicare generally does not cover ongoing custodial care.

It is important to understand early that while in-home care can feel more manageable at first, it may not always be the most cost-effective solution once 24/7 supervision becomes necessary.

Benefits

Families often choose in-home care because:

- Your loved one stays in familiar surroundings
- Routines feel less disrupted
- There is more privacy and autonomy
- Care can start gradually
- It feels like a softer transition than moving

For many people in the earlier or middle stages of dementia, this option can provide meaningful support while preserving routine.

It can also allow family members to shift from being the only caregiver to being part of a caregiving team.

That shift alone can change everything.

Limitations

In-home care is not without challenges.

- Care is only present during scheduled hours. If wandering, falls, or nighttime confusion are increasing, gaps in supervision can become risky.
- Care coordination often falls to the family — scheduling, communication, monitoring, and adjusting services.
- Consistency can vary depending on staffing.
- And as needs increase, so do costs.

It's also important to acknowledge something gently but honestly:

Even with professional support, family members often remain emotionally "on call." Bringing in help does not automatically eliminate stress — it redistributes it.

When In-Home Care Works Best

In-home care often works well when:

- Your loved one is still relatively mobile
- Nighttime supervision is not yet critical
- Behavioral symptoms are manageable
- The home environment is safe
- The primary caregiver needs structured relief

It can also serve as a transitional step — a way to assess needs more clearly before considering memory care or skilled nursing.

Choosing in-home care does not lock you into that choice forever. It is one chapter in a longer journey.

Quick Guide: How to Choose an In-Home Care Agency

1. Basics You Should Never Skip

☐ Is the agency **licensed** in your state?

☐ Are caregivers **employees** (not independent contractors)?

☐ Does the agency carry **liability insurance & workers' comp**?

☐ Are background checks and drug screens required?

If an agency hesitates or dodges these questions, that's your answer.

2. Training & Dementia Experience

☐ What **dementia-specific training** do caregivers receive?

☐ How often is training updated?

☐ Are caregivers trained to handle:

- agitation or sundowning
- falls or near-falls
- wandering
- resistance to care

☐ Is there a **care supervisor or nurse** you can contact if something goes wrong?

3. Consistency & Staffing Reality

☐ Will you have **consistent caregivers**, or frequent rotation?

☐ What happens if your caregiver calls out sick?

☐ Can the agency provide **backup coverage** quickly?

☐ Are overnight or weekend hours available if needs increase?

This is where expectations vs. reality matter *a lot.*

4. Safety & Communication

☐ How are **care notes documented** and shared with family?

☐ How are **changes in condition** communicated?

☐ Who do you call in an emergency — and after hours?

☐ How do they handle **falls or incidents**?

A gentle reminder: You are not being difficult by asking these questions. You are being responsible.

5. Scope of Care & Boundaries

☐ What **they will and will not do** (very important)

☐ Medication reminders vs. administration

☐ Mobility and transfer assistance

☐ Toileting and bathing support

☐ Meal prep vs. feeding assistance

This prevents heartbreak later when assumptions collide with policy.

6. Costs & Contracts

☐ Hourly rate and minimum hours

☐ Overtime, holiday, or overnight rates

☐ Cancellation policies

☐ Rate increases as care needs change

☐ What long-term care insurance *will* and *won't* reimburse

Get everything in writing. Even the things you hope won't change.

7. The Gut Check (Underrated but Crucial)

☐ Do they listen without rushing you?

☐ Do they speak respectfully about people with dementia?

☐ Do you feel pressured to decide quickly?

☐ Do you feel relief — even a little — after the conversation?

That last one matters more than people realize.

When Home Is No Longer the Safest Place

There is no single moment that signals it's time to consider a facility—but there are patterns that deserve attention.

You may notice:

- Frequent falls or injuries
- Increasing agitation or unsafe behaviors
- Wandering or nighttime disruption
- Medical needs you can't manage at home
- Your own health is declining
- Constant fear of "what might happen next."

These are not signs you're failing. They are signs that care needs have outgrown what one person can safely provide.

A Financial Reality You're Not Imagining

This is often where guilt intensifies—because even when caregivers *know* they can't safely do it alone, options feel limited.

Financial Reality Check: Insurance, Medicaid, and Hard Limits

Many caregivers quietly believe that if they just try harder, sacrifice more, or stretch themselves further, they'll be able to make everything work.

The reality is that dementia care is expensive, and most families are navigating **limitations**, not choices.

Long-term care insurance, when available, can help—but coverage varies, benefits may be capped, and delays are common.

Medicare does not cover long-term custodial care. This often comes as a shock.

Without long-term care insurance, families are often choosing between:

- Paying privately until resources are exhausted
- Relying on unpaid family caregiving
- Exploring **Medicaid-supported facilities or services**

Medicaid facilities vary widely and often require extensive documentation and waiting periods. Choosing Medicaid-supported care is not "giving up." It is using the system that exists when other options aren't available.

Loving someone does not erase practical limits.

What to Expect Emotionally When You Consider Placement

Even when placement is clearly needed, the emotional response can be intense.

Caregivers often feel:

- Guilt for needing help
- Fear of judgment
- Grief over another loss of a role
- Relief mixed with shame

All of these emotions can coexist. Relief does not mean you didn't love them enough. It means the load was heavy.

A Caregiver's Voice

Please do not ask your loved one whether they want to go to a safer place, facility, memory care, or assisted living. You will not get the response you hope for. I chose not to tell my mom we were going into a facility until move-in day and said we were going to a new home. I took her clothes, toiletries, photos, and items with sentimental value. I told her we were moving there. We were doing it together. I'm not gonna lie. Leaving her there that day was awful and probably the hardest thing I had to do to that point in my life. But if you've done your homework, you've found caregivers who are skilled at helping new residents adjust. The next couple of weeks are going to be awful for you, and I'm so sorry you're going to go through this. In the in-between moments, however, you may start to feel a little lighter and more hopeful knowing that your loved one is being well cared for—in some cases, more informed care than they got at home.

Researching Memory Care and Skilled Facilities

If you begin exploring facilities, take your time when possible. I've included a basic facility checklist at the end of this chapter that you can make copies of as you visit facilities in the area.

Consider:

- Staff training and staff-to-patient ratios
- How agitation or behavioral issues are handled
- Medical oversight and emergency protocols
- Daily routines and structure
- Activities available to maintain mental stimulation
- What daily living activities do they handle? Are there any they do not?
- Safety features
- Cost transparency
- Is the memory care unit secure?

Ask directly how they handle falls, infections, aggression, and end-of-life care. You are not being difficult—you are being responsible.

What to Take to a Facility

Bringing familiar items can ease transition:

- Photos
- Favorite blankets or clothing
- Small furniture pieces (if allowed); note that some facilities may require you to furnish the room. Be sure to cover this in your initial visit with the facility and director.
- Music or personal objects

Familiarity can reduce anxiety, even when memory is impaired.

A Decision Checklist: Is It Time to Consider a Facility?

You don't need to check every box. One may be enough to deserve serious attention.

- I no longer feel my loved one is safe at home
- I am afraid of what might happen when I'm not there
- My physical or mental health is suffering
- Medical or behavioral needs exceed my ability to manage
- Injuries or near-misses are becoming more frequent
- Care has become 24/7 with no relief
- Waiting feels more dangerous than acting

If you checked any of these, it doesn't mean you must place your loved one now. It means the question deserves serious attention.

In Closing

There is no single right choice in this chapter—only the right choice for your family, your resources, and your loved one's current needs. Decisions about care are shaped by finances, insurance coverage, geography, available services, family dynamics, and the specific way dementia is unfolding. What feels possible for one family may be impossible for another. Comparison will only add weight you don't need to carry.

What matters most is safety, dignity, and sustainability—for everyone involved.

- You are not choosing "the end" — you are choosing support
- This chapter is a snapshot, not a verdict
- Encouragement to trust observation over fear

- Permission to revisit, reassess, and adjust

Reflection Prompts

You don't need to answer every question. Some are meant to sit with you rather than be solved.

Examining Beliefs About Care

- What messages have I internalized about what a "good" caregiver should do?
- Where did the belief that I *have* to do this myself come from?
- How has that belief helped me—and how has it harmed me?

Safety vs. Guilt

- Am I making decisions based more on guilt or on safety?
- What risks am I carrying that feel unsustainable?
- If someone I loved were in my position, what would I want for them?

Acknowledging Limits

- What parts of caregiving now feel beyond my training, strength, or capacity?
- What would it mean to accept that love has limits—but responsibility doesn't have to be solitary?
- What signs tell me that waiting may be more dangerous than acting?

Financial Reality

- What financial constraints are shaping my options right now?
- Have I been blaming myself for systemic limitations?
- What would it feel like to make the *best possible* decision within real-world limits?

Redefining Care

- If caregiving changes form, how might my role change rather than disappear?
- What parts of care—advocacy, presence, love—will always remain mine?
- What does dignity look like for my loved one at this stage?

A Gentle Reminder

Needing more help does not mean you love them less. It means their needs have grown bigger than one person can safely hold.

Choosing a facility is not walking away from caregiving. It is changing where and how you care, so that safety, dignity, and connection can be shared.

Guilt will tell you that a "good" caregiver would keep going no matter the cost. Wisdom—and love—recognize when the cost has become too high for everyone.

Looking Ahead

Placement doesn't end caregiving—it changes it.

In the next chapter, we'll talk about what life looks like *after* placement: how to stay involved, advocate effectively, and maintain connection even when care is shared with others.

Facility Comparison Worksheet

Use this worksheet to compare a few options side by side. You are not looking for perfection—you are looking for patterns of safety, respect, and fit.

Facility Name: _______________________________________

Location: _______________________________________

Type: ☐ Memory Care ☐ Skilled Nursing ☐ Other
Cost (monthly): __________

<u>Staffing & Training</u>

- Staff-to-resident ratio: __________________
- Dementia-specific training? ☐ Yes ☐ No ☐ Unclear
- Consistent staff or frequent turnover? ________

<u>Medical & Safety</u>

- On-site medical staff? ☐ Yes ☐ No
- How are falls handled? __________________
- How are infections or sudden changes addressed?

- Emergency protocols explained clearly? ☐ Yes ☐ No

<u>Behavior & Emotional Care</u>

- How is agitation handled? ________________
- Are medications used as a first response? ☐ Yes ☐ No

- How is sundowning managed?

  ____

- How are residents redirected or comforted?

  ____

Daily Life

- Structured routines? ☐ Yes ☐ No
- Activities appropriate for dementia?

  ____

- Opportunities for calm and rest? ☐ Yes ☐ No
- Clean, calm environment? _______________

Family Involvement

- Are visiting hours flexible? ☐ Yes ☐ No
- Encouraged to visit at different times? ☐ Yes ☐ No
- Is communication with family clear and regular? ___
- How are concerns handled?

  ____

End-of-Life & Transitions

- Hospice allowed on-site? ☐ Yes ☐ No
- How do they handle decline or end-of-life care?

  ____

Overall Impressions

- Did staff speak respectfully about residents? ☐ Yes ☐ No
- Did I feel rushed or welcomed?

  ____

- What felt right here?

____

____

- What gave me pause?

____

After Visiting

- Could I imagine my loved one being safe here?
- Could *I* imagine being supported as a family member?
- What questions remain unanswered?

Chapter 9 — Life in a Facility

If you're reading this chapter, you've crossed one of the hardest thresholds of caregiving.

Life in Memory Care: What It Is — and What It Isn't

For many caregivers, moving a loved one into memory care brings a complicated sense of relief. After months or years of carrying the responsibility alone, it can feel like exhaling for the first time in a long while.

There is comfort in knowing your loved one is no longer at home alone, no longer wandering outside, no longer relying solely on your vigilance to stay safe.

That relief is real. And deserved.

But it's also important to understand what memory care *actually* provides — and what it doesn't — so you're not left with a false sense of security or unnecessary guilt when reality doesn't match expectations.

Memory care is a shared-care environment. It is designed to support safety, dignity, and routine — **not to eliminate all risk** or replace family advocacy.

Knowing this ahead of time doesn't make the transition harder.

It makes it healthier.

A Shared Environment, Not One-on-One Care

Memory care units are typically secure, enclosed spaces designed to allow residents to move freely within safe boundaries. Residents are usually encouraged to walk, explore, and remain mobile for as long as possible.

This means:

- Your loved one may walk independently within the unit
- They may enter common areas or other residents' spaces
- Staff cannot — and should not — keep eyes on any one person at all times

This isn't a flaw in the system. It's a conscious design choice meant to preserve autonomy and reduce agitation.

At the same time, it requires families to adjust expectations. Memory care is **supervised**, not individualized minute-by-minute.

Why Belongings Sometimes Go Missing

One of the first surprises many families encounter is missing personal items.

Glasses disappear. Blankets wander. Books, sweaters, framed photos — even shoes — can turn up in someone else's room.

This usually isn't theft.

It's recognition confusion.

Residents may genuinely believe an item belongs to them, or that they've had it forever. Labeling items helps, but it won't prevent this entirely. *(Personal note: I put my mom's last name and room number on just about everything. It's especially recommended for anything that goes to laundry to reduce loss.)*

The emotional impact can be bigger than expected. Personal items feel like extensions of identity — especially when so much else has already been lost.

Knowing this is common can soften that first wave of frustration or hurt.

Staffing Realities — Even in Excellent Facilities

Even the best memory care facilities operate with limited staff relative to resident needs. Staff members are assisting multiple residents at once, rotating through routines, responding to needs as they arise.

This means:

- Care is responsive, not constant
- Staff may not witness every incident
- Some changes are noticed gradually, not immediately

This is not negligence. It's the reality of communal care.

Families often assume that once a loved one enters memory care, oversight becomes complete. In reality, **family involvement remains an essential layer of care**.

A Caregiver's Voice

I love the facility that my mom is in. I did hours and hours of research. But a facility can look great during a visit and say all the right things, and you still find that they're not what you'd hoped for. This is my mom's second facility, and involved a move for us both from North Carolina to Florida.

I visit at all different times and days of the week to get a feel for the staff, and to assess care on different shifts. I remember visiting one day, and I found myself alone in a big living room with about 12 patients, including my mom. Thank goodness, nothing happened, but the potential risk was enough for me to talk with the Director of Nursing and the Executive Director. I had compiled a list of questions by the time I scheduled the meeting. I found them to be professional and appropriate, and most importantly, I think they appreciated knowing the areas that needed attention. Advocacy doesn't end with placement.

Falls: A Difficult but Common Reality

Falls are one of the hardest things for families to accept — and one of the most common realities in memory care.

Dementia affects:

- Balance
- Depth perception
- Judgment
- Awareness of physical limits

Even in well-designed environments with attentive staff, falls happen.

A fall does not automatically mean something went wrong.

It does not mean you made the wrong decision.

It does not mean the facility failed.

The goal of memory care is **risk reduction**, not risk elimination — while preserving dignity and mobility as long as possible.

Cameras, Monitoring, and Peace of Mind

Some facilities have fall-detection systems or room monitoring in place. Others do not.

It's reasonable to ask:

- Are cameras or monitoring systems already in use?
- Are personal cameras allowed in private rooms?
- What consent rules apply if there is a roommate?

If cameras are permitted, they can provide reassurance — especially during the early adjustment period.

They should be used as a **support tool**, not a source of constant vigilance or anxiety. Trust, communication, and relationship-building with staff matter just as much.

Advocacy Doesn't End — It Evolves

Placing a loved one in memory care does not mean stepping away.

It means stepping into a different role. *(See Glossary: Palliative Care and Hospice)*

Advocacy in this phase isn't about control. It's about collaboration.

You are no longer the sole caregiver — but you are still the most consistent voice for your loved one's history, preferences, and needs.

Quick Reality Check

Memory Care Provides:

- A secured environment
- Structured routines
- Trained dementia-aware staff
- Reduced isolation

Memory Care Does Not Guarantee:

- One-on-one supervision
- No falls or injuries
- No missing items
- Perfect communication
- The end of advocacy

Understanding this difference protects you from guilt, anger, and unrealistic expectations.

Quick Guide: One-Page Advocacy Checklist

(A practical guide for staying engaged without burning out)

Build Relationships

- Learn staff members' names
- Be respectful and appreciative
- Approach concerns as shared problem-solving

Communicate What Matters

- Share your loved one's routines, triggers, comforts, and history
- Speak up early when something feels "off"
- Ask questions — calmly and consistently

Stay Observant, Not Hypervigilant

- Visit at varied times if possible
- Notice patterns rather than isolated moments
- Document recurring concerns

Prepare for Common Challenges

- Label belongings
- Expect occasional missing items
- Understand fall protocols and reporting processes

Use Tools Wisely

- Ask about monitoring or camera policies
- Use technology for reassurance, not surveillance
- Keep communication lines open with staff

Protect Yourself

- Set realistic expectations
- Accept what no system can fully control
- Remember: placement was an act of care, not abandonment

Now that you have a clearer picture of what memory care is — and what it isn't — it's time to talk about what happens next. The first week after placement is often the most emotionally charged for both caregivers and their loved ones. Even when the decision was necessary and thoughtfully made, this period can bring waves of doubt, grief, relief, and second-guessing. What you're about to experience isn't a sign that something is wrong — it's a normal part of transition. Understanding what the first week may look like can help you move through it with steadiness rather than fear.

The First Week After Placement: What to Expect

If you've just placed your loved one in a facility and feel shaken, guilty, or unsure you did the right thing—start here.

The first week after placement is often harder on caregivers than it is on the person with dementia. You may feel heartache and overwhelming sadness, be disoriented, feel emotionally raw, or be haunted by second-guessing. That doesn't mean placement was a mistake. It means you're grieving another change in role.

The facility may encourage you to wait a week or two before coming back to visit. This is for both you and your loved one. It's very likely that your loved one will experience increased agitation, fear, and sadness. It's incredibly hard on the caregiver to process this level of pain and fear. It can break even the strongest and most stoic individuals. But it gets better. They will adjust to the staff and learn the new routines. And the staff needs to learn about your loved one as well. So if they ask you to give it time before returning, give it serious consideration.

Here's what many caregivers experience during that first week—and why it's normal.

Quick Guide: In the First Days After Placement

You don't have to get everything right in the first week. Aim small.

- Expect mixed emotions in you: grief, guilt, relief, anger, numbness—they can all show up on the same day.

- Expect your loved one to seem "worse" at times: more confused, fearful, or withdrawn. This often reflects transition, not failure.

- Ask one staff member to be your main point of contact, if possible, so you're not telling your story over and over.

- Keep visits shorter and calmer at first, unless staff suggest otherwise. Watch how your loved one does during and after visits.

- Jot down questions or concerns after each visit, and bring them to the nurse or care team instead of trying to fix everything on the spot.

Emotional Whiplash Is Common

You may feel relief one moment and crushing guilt the next. You may miss your loved one intensely while also feeling physically lighter. These emotions can coexist without canceling each other out.

Relief does not mean you failed. It means the burden was heavy.

Your Loved One May Seem "Worse"

It's common for people with dementia to appear more confused, withdrawn, or agitated during the first days or weeks. New environments, unfamiliar routines, and sensory changes take time to adjust to.

This does not mean the facility is not doing enough or is bad. It means transition is happening.

Visiting Patterns Matter

In the first week, shorter, calmer visits are often better than long, emotionally charged ones. Watch your loved one's cues. Some people settle more easily when visits are consistent but not overwhelming.

There is no single "right" approach—only what reduces distress.

Staff Are Still Learning About Your Loved One

You know your loved one better than anyone. Staff need time to learn routines, preferences, and triggers. This is normal. It's also why your input matters early.

Advocacy doesn't stop at placement—it changes form.

Life After the First Week

Once the initial shock begins to settle, caregiving becomes a shared responsibility. This shift can feel disorienting.

You are no longer responsible for every task—but you are still essential.

Visiting Often And at Different Times

If possible, visit at varying times of day. This gives you a more accurate picture of care and helps you notice patterns.

Your presence:

- Signals continued involvement
- Builds relationships with staff
- Helps identify issues early

You don't need to hover. Consistent presence is enough.

Advocating Without Undermining Care

Advocacy in a facility is about collaboration, not confrontation.

Helpful approaches include:

- Sharing insights about preferences and triggers
- Asking questions respectfully and directly
- Documenting concerns and follow-ups
- Requesting care plan meetings when needed

You are part of the care team—even when care is no longer solely yours.

When Injuries or Issues Occur in a Facility

Falls, infections, and incidents still happen in facilities. Placement reduces risk—it does not eliminate it.

When something occurs:

- Ask for a clear explanation

- Request documentation
- Monitor patterns
- Escalate concerns when necessary

Trust your instincts. If something feels off, follow up.

Maintaining Connection When Communication Changes

Even as verbal communication fades, connection remains possible.

Connection may come through:

- Sitting quietly
- Music or familiar objects
- Gentle touch (when welcomed)
- Shared routines

Your presence still matters—even when words don't.

A Caregiver's Voice

Leaving my Mom at the facility the first day was gut-wrenching. But the staff was skilled at redirection, and her attention was diverted to more pleasant thoughts. However, the first week after placement nearly broke me. Watching my Mom be emotionally hurt and scared was more than my heart could take. I didn't wait for the suggested time and learned my lesson the hard way. However, the next visit was better, and the good news was that my Mom didn't remember that awful evening.

Reflection Prompts

You don't need to answer all of these. Some are meant simply to be read and felt.

- ☐ What feelings come up most often when I leave the facility—relief, guilt, sadness, anger, something else?

- ☐ How has my role as a caregiver changed since placement—and what parts of care still clearly belong to me?

- ☐ When I visit, what seems to comfort my loved one the most (time of day, length of visit, activities, tone)?

- ☐ What patterns have I noticed about the facility—times when care seems strong, and times when I need to speak up more?

- ☐ How can I build a working relationship with staff that feels collaborative rather than adversarial?

- ☐ What helps me remember that advocating for better care is not the same as attacking the people providing it?

A Gentle Reminder

Placement changes the tasks you do, but it does not erase your importance. You are still your loved one's historian, advocate, and source of familiar love.

There will be days when you question the decision and days when you feel deep relief. Both are honest responses, not verdicts on your worth.

You are allowed to let the facility carry some of the weight while you focus on what only you can offer: presence, memory, and care that comes from knowing them by heart.

Looking Ahead

Life in a facility brings new rhythms—and new questions. As dementia progresses, attention often turns toward comfort, dignity, and what the final stages may look like.

In the next chapter, we'll talk about late-stage dementia, hospice, and how to know when the focus shifts from treatment to comfort—and how to walk that path with compassion.

Chapter 10 — The Final Stages and End of Life

There comes a point in dementia caregiving when the questions change.

Instead of *How do we manage this?* Or what *comes next?* Caregivers begin asking quieter, heavier questions:

- *How much longer can this go on?*
- *Are they comfortable?*
- *Am I doing the right things now?*

This chapter is not about predicting timelines. Dementia does not follow a calendar. It's about understanding what changes as the disease advances—and how to respond with compassion, clarity, and presence.

What Late-Stage Dementia Often Looks Like

In the later stages of dementia, the body and brain gradually slow down.

Caregivers may notice:

- Significant memory loss, including recognition of loved ones
- Limited or absent verbal communication
- Increased sleeping
- Difficulty swallowing or eating
- Weight loss and physical frailty
- Reduced mobility or complete dependence
- Changes in breathing or alertness

These changes can be deeply distressing to witness. They often arrive gradually, but the cumulative effect can feel overwhelming.

It's important to remember: these changes are caused by the disease—not by anything you did or failed to do.

What the End of Life Often Looks Like in Dementia

Common Physical Changes

- Increased sleeping (sometimes most of the day)
- Decreased appetite and eventual loss of interest in food
- Difficulty swallowing (choking risk, aspiration)
- Weight loss and muscle wasting
- Less mobility → bedbound
- Changes in breathing patterns near the very end

Common Cognitive / Behavioral Changes

- Minimal or absent speech
- Less eye contact or responsiveness
- Periods of agitation alternating with long calm
- Reaching, picking, or repetitive motions
- Apparent "withdrawal" that is neurological, not emotional

Emotional Reality for Caregivers

- Feeling like they are "disappearing before death."
- Fear that stopping food or treatment is "giving up."
- Distress when a loved one no longer recognizes them
- Confusion about whether pain is present

- These changes are **not caused by a lack of care**
- Reduced eating is part of the dying process, not starvation
- Comfort-focused care often *reduces* suffering
- Dementia itself is a terminal illness — many caregivers are never told this

The Lived Reality of Dying with Dementia

One of the hardest parts of this journey is that many caregivers are never told what dying *from* dementia can look like. Without that context, normal changes can feel alarming—like something is going wrong, or something important is being missed.

In reality, dementia is a terminal illness, and the end of life often unfolds gradually.

As the body and brain slow down, caregivers may notice that their loved one sleeps more—sometimes most of the day. Appetite often decreases, then fades altogether. Eating can become difficult or unsafe as swallowing reflexes weaken, increasing the risk of choking or aspiration. Weight loss and physical frailty are common, even when care is attentive and loving.

These changes are not caused by a lack of care. They are part of the body's natural shutting-down process.

Communication often becomes limited or disappears entirely. Your loved one may no longer respond in familiar ways, make eye contact, or seem aware of who is present. This can feel like another profound loss—especially when recognition is gone.

What looks like emotional withdrawal is neurological, not a reflection of love or connection.

Some patients experience periods of restlessness or agitation near the end, while others grow increasingly calm. You may notice repetitive movements, reaching, picking at blankets, or quiet vocalizations. These behaviors are common and do not necessarily indicate pain or distress, though they should always be assessed and addressed for comfort.

Caregivers often struggle most when eating stops. It can feel deeply wrong—like starvation, like giving up, like causing harm. In truth, loss of appetite is a natural part of the dying process. Forcing food or fluids at this stage can cause more discomfort, not less. Comfort-focused care prioritizes easing symptoms rather than prolonging bodily functions that are already slowing.

Breathing patterns may also change in the final phase, becoming irregular or shallow. These changes can be unsettling to witness, even when your loved one appears peaceful.

Perhaps the most painful reality is that many caregivers feel they are losing their loved one before death occurs. This ambiguous loss—grieving someone who is still alive—can feel unbearable. If you find yourself mourning while still showing up each day, know that this is a natural response to a long goodbye.

Nothing about this stage means you failed. Nothing here suggests you should have done more. Being present, ensuring comfort, and allowing the body to do what it needs to do are not abandonment—they are care.

Shifting the Focus: From Treatment to Comfort

Earlier in the journey, caregiving often centers on managing symptoms, preventing decline, and responding to crises. In the final stages, the focus shifts.

The primary questions become:

- Are they comfortable?
- Are they safe?
- Are they at peace?

Comfort-focused care, sometimes called palliative care, prioritizes relief from pain, anxiety, breathlessness, and distress. It values dignity and quality of life over prolonging life at all costs.

This shift can feel emotionally complex. Choosing comfort does not mean choosing less care. It means choosing different care.

Transitioning: The Act of Dying

As dementia reaches its final stage, there is often a period referred to as transitioning or active dying. This phase can be deeply emotional for caregivers, especially when they are unsure what changes are normal.

During this time, caregivers may notice:

- Long periods of unresponsiveness
- Minimal interest in food or fluids
- Changes in breathing patterns
- Coolness in hands or feet
- Less engagement with surroundings

These changes are part of the body's natural process of slowing down and shutting down. They are not usually painful, even though they can be difficult to witness.

This phase is often quieter than earlier stages. The work of caregiving becomes less about doing and more about being— offering comfort, presence, and calm.

If hospice is involved, the team can help interpret what you're seeing and manage symptoms. If it's not, you can still ask providers what signs to expect so you're not left guessing.

Transitioning is not something to fix or stop. It is something to accompany.

How Do You Know When It's Time for Hospice?

Many caregivers worry that bringing in hospice means "giving up." In reality, hospice is about **support** for both the person with dementia and the people who love them.

Hospice may be appropriate when:

- Dementia has progressed to advanced stages
- Your loved one is no longer benefiting from curative treatments
- There has been a significant functional decline
- Eating and swallowing have become difficult
- Infections or hospitalizations are frequent
- The focus has shifted toward comfort

Hospice teams typically include nurses, aides, social workers, chaplains, and physicians. They help manage symptoms, provide guidance, and support caregivers through one of the hardest phases of the journey.

Importantly, hospice does not mean care stops. It means care becomes more intentional and supportive.

Quick Guide: Questions to Ask When End of Life Is Near

You don't need to know all the right questions. These can be a starting point with hospice or the care team:

Comfort and symptoms

- How will you keep them comfortable if pain, shortness of breath, or agitation increases?
- What signs should I call you about right away?

Interventions and decisions

- At this stage, what treatments are likely to help—and which might only prolong suffering?
- How will we decide when to stop certain tests, transfers, or hospital trips?

My role

- What can I do at the bedside that is actually helpful—for them and for you?
- Are there times when it's better for me to rest and let staff take over?

The road ahead

- ☐ What changes might I see in the coming days or weeks?
- ☐ How will I know when we are very close to the end?

Writing these down and bringing them to a meeting can make an impossible conversation a little more manageable.

What Hospice Can Offer Caregivers

Hospice care often brings relief that caregivers didn't realize they needed.

It can provide:

- Regular nursing visits
- On-call support for urgent concerns
- Medication management focused on comfort
- Equipment and supplies
- Emotional and spiritual support
- Guidance through the dying process

Many caregivers later say they wish hospice had been involved sooner.

Letting Go of "Doing Enough"

As the end approaches, caregivers often struggle with guilt—wondering if they should be doing more, trying harder, or intervening differently.

This is one of the most painful parts of the journey.

At this stage, *doing enough* often looks like:

- Being present
- Providing comfort
- Speaking gently
- Advocating for dignity
- Allowing rest

You do not need to fight the disease to love the person.

Being Present When Words Are Gone

Even when communication is minimal or absent, presence still matters.

Your loved one may still respond to:

- Familiar voices
- Gentle touch (when welcomed)
- Music
- Calm energy

You don't need to say the perfect thing. Simply being there is enough.

Reflection Prompts

You may not have the energy to answer these fully. Reading them is enough.

- ☐ What fears do I carry about being present at the end of my loved one's life?

- ☐ When I think about "doing enough," whose voice am I hearing—mine, my loved one's, family, culture, faith?

- What would it look like to measure my care in terms of comfort, presence, and love rather than medical heroics?

- Are there words I want to say, or moments I hope to share, while there is still time—even if they can't fully respond?

- How can I build in small rests or support for myself during this time, knowing that my body and mind are under extreme strain?

- If a close friend were in my place, what would I tell them about what "enough" looks like at the end of life?

A Gentle Reminder

There is no perfect way to walk someone you love to the edge of their life. There are only imperfect moments of presence, care, and love.

Medical choices at the end of life are rarely clear-cut. Whatever decisions you make, you are making them inside grief, exhaustion, and uncertainty—not from indifference.

The fact that you are worrying about "doing enough" is itself evidence of your love. You are allowed to choose comfort over prolonging suffering, and to trust that love is measured in presence, not in perfection.

Looking Ahead

The end of life does not mark the end of grief. For caregivers, loss often continues long after caregiving responsibilities have ended.

In the final chapter, we'll talk about what comes after—ongoing grief, rebuilding identity, and carrying love forward after years of caregiving and loss.

Hospice Decision Checklist

This checklist isn't about certainty. It's about noticing patterns and giving yourself permission to ask for support.

You don't need to check every box.

Changes in Your Loved One

- ☐ Significant decline in physical strength or mobility
- ☐ Eating and swallowing have become difficult or unsafe
- ☐ Increased sleeping or decreased responsiveness
- ☐ Frequent infections or hospitalizations
- ☐ Limited or no verbal communication
- ☐ Signs of discomfort, pain, anxiety, or agitation

Changes in Care Goals

- ☐ Treatments no longer improve the quality of life
- ☐ The focus feels more like comfort than recovery
- ☐ Hospital visits feel burdensome rather than helpful
- ☐ You are questioning whether continued interventions are kind

Caregiver Experience

- ☐ I feel overwhelmed by managing symptoms alone
- ☐ I need guidance about what to expect next

☐   I want support that includes emotional care for me

☐   I feel afraid of making the wrong decision

Practical Indicators

☐   A healthcare provider has mentioned hospice

☐   I am unsure how much time may be left

☐   I need help managing medications, equipment, or comfort care

If You Checked Any of These

It may be time to **ask about hospice**, even if you're not ready to decide.

Asking does not commit you to anything. Hospice can be:

- A consultation
- An added layer of support
- A source of guidance during uncertainty

Many families say they waited longer than necessary.

Chapter 11 — After and Ongoing Grief

When caregiving ends, many people expect the pain to end with it.

Instead, grief often changes shape.

For caregivers, loss does not arrive all at once. It has been unfolding for years—quietly, repeatedly, and without ceremony. By the time death occurs, you may feel emptied out, numb, or strangely unmoored. Others may expect you to "move on," not realizing how much you have already lost—and how much you are still losing.

This chapter is about what happens *after* dementia caregiving ends—and why grief doesn't follow a tidy timeline.

Grief After Dementia Is Different

Dementia grief is layered.

You may grieve:

- The person your loved one was before the disease
- The years spent caregiving
- The version of yourself shaped by responsibility
- The life you put on hold
- The relief you feel—and the guilt that may follow it

Some caregivers are surprised to find that the grief after death feels quieter than expected. Others are overwhelmed by a delayed wave of sorrow once the constant vigilance stops.

There is no correct response.

When Caregiving Ends, Identity Often Shifts

For a long time, caregiving structured your days, decisions, and sense of purpose. When it ends, you may feel untethered.

You might ask:

- *Who am I without this role?*
- *What do I do with my time now?*
- *Why do I feel lost when I should feel free?*

This loss of identity is real—and rarely acknowledged. Rebuilding a sense of self takes time, patience, and gentleness.

You don't need to reinvent yourself immediately. Rest is allowed.

Quick Guide: In the First Weeks After Caregiving Ends

You do not need a life plan right now. Think in days, not years.

Keep decisions small

- ☐ Delay big life changes (selling homes, major moves, big commitments) if you can.

- ☐ Focus on the next few weeks, not the rest of your life.

Tend to your body

- ☐ Notice sleep, appetite, and pain.

☐ Schedule at least one basic medical or therapy check-in for yourself when you're able.

Choose one "anchor" each day

☐ A short walk, a shower, a meal, a phone call, a small creative act—something that marks the day as yours too.

Let support in, a little at a time

☐ Say yes to specific offers that truly help (a meal, company at an appointment, help with paperwork).

☐ If people say "Let me know if you need anything," consider naming one small, concrete thing.

You are recovering from years of hypervigilance. Rest is not laziness; it is repair.

Relief and Guilt Can Coexist

Many caregivers feel relief when their loved one is no longer suffering—and then feel ashamed for feeling it.

Relief does not cancel love.

Relief does not diminish grief.

Relief does not mean you wanted the loss.

It means the suffering ended—for both of you.

Grief Is Not Linear

Some days will feel manageable. Others may knock the wind out of you without warning. Anniversaries, songs, smells, or moments of quiet can unexpectedly reopen grief.

This does not mean you're going backward. It means grief moves in waves.

Allow the waves. They lessen over time.

Carrying Memories Without Carrying Pain

For many caregivers, memories are complicated. Some are tender. Others are painful. You may struggle to remember who your loved one was before the disease without also remembering who they became.

Over time, many people find that memories soften. The disease loosens its grip on the narrative, and earlier moments re-emerge.

You don't need to force this process. It unfolds naturally, in its own time.

Finding Support After Caregiving Ends

When caregiving ends, support often disappears—just when it's still needed.

You may benefit from:

- Grief counseling or therapy
- Caregiver bereavement groups
- Journaling or creative expression
- Rituals of remembrance
- Reconnecting slowly with interests or community

There is no deadline for grief. You are allowed to take up space with it.

Meaning After Loss

Meaning does not come from suffering itself. It comes from how you carry what you've lived through.

Many caregivers discover:

- Increased compassion for others
- A deeper understanding of vulnerability
- A clearer sense of what matters

You don't need to turn pain into purpose to justify it. If meaning emerges, let it. If it doesn't, that's okay too.

Reflection Prompts

You may want to return to these over time. Grief changes—and so will your answers.

After Caregiving Ends

- What feels most different now that caregiving has ended?
- In what moments do I feel untethered, quiet, or unsure of who I am?
- What parts of caregiving do I miss—even if I don't miss the responsibility?

Grief Without a Timeline

- ☐ How does grief show up for me right now—emotionally, physically, or mentally?
- ☐ Are there moments when grief catches me off guard?
- ☐ What expectations—mine or others'—feel heavy or unrealistic?

Relief, Love, and Guilt

- ☐ Have I experienced relief alongside grief?
- ☐ What feelings have I judged myself for?
- ☐ What would it sound like to allow these emotions to coexist without explanation?

Carrying Memories Forward

- ☐ What memories feel hardest to hold right now?
- ☐ Are there moments I want to remember apart from the disease?
- ☐ How might I honor my loved one in a way that feels authentic to me?

Meaning After Loss

- ☐ What, if anything, has caregiving changed in how I see myself or others?
- ☐ Where do I notice even a small sense of clarity about what matters to me now?

☐ Do I feel any pull—however faint—toward something that feels like life after this?

A Gentle Reminder

You do not have to "move on" from someone you loved. You need to go on. You are learning how to go on while carrying what you've lived through.

There is no right pace for grief after dementia. Numbness, anger, relief, deep sadness, or even moments of unexpected lightness— all of them belong.

The years you spent caring have changed you, but they do not have to define all of who you are. You are allowed to rest, to rebuild, and to imagine a life that holds both what you've lost and what is still possible.

A Closing Thought

If you have made it this far—through uncertainty, exhaustion, heartbreak, and loss—know this:

You loved deeply. You showed up repeatedly. You did the best you could in an impossible situation.

Grief may walk with you for a while longer. But it does not erase the love, the care, the advocacy, or the presence you gave.

Those things remain.

Appendix A — Glossary of Terms

This glossary is here for reference, not mastery.

You don't need to memorize these terms or understand them all at once.

Use this section when a word feels unfamiliar or overwhelming—and then return to the page you were on.

ADLs (Activities of Daily Living)

A term used by healthcare providers to describe basic self-care tasks that allow a person to function independently.

ADLs often include:

- Bathing and personal hygiene
- Dressing
- Eating
- Toileting
- Transferring (moving from bed to chair, standing, walking)
- Continence

In dementia care, changes in ADLs are often more meaningful than memory test scores. Difficulty with ADLs helps providers assess disease progression, care needs, and eligibility for services such as home care, memory care, long-term care insurance benefits, or hospice.

Loss of ADL independence is neurological—not a lack of effort or cooperation.

Advance Directives / Living Will

Legal documents that outline a person's wishes for medical care
if they are unable to communicate those wishes themselves,
particularly near the end of life.

Agitation

Restlessness, anxiety, irritability, or emotional distress that may
show up as pacing, anger, resistance, or repetitive behaviors.
Often a sign of unmet needs rather than intentional behavior.

Alzheimer's Disease

The most common cause of dementia. It primarily affects
memory early on but eventually impacts thinking, behavior, and
physical function.

Anosognosia

A neurological condition in which a person is unable to recognize
or understand their own illness or impairments. This is not
denial or stubbornness—it's caused by changes in the brain.

Anticipatory Grief

Grief that occurs before death is often experienced by caregivers
as they witness ongoing losses while their loved one is still alive.

Apathy

A common symptom of dementia is marked by reduced
motivation, interest, or emotional responsiveness. Apathy may

look like indifference, withdrawal, lack of initiative, or seeming "checked out."

Apathy is not laziness, depression, or lack of caring. It is caused by changes in the brain that affect motivation and emotional processing.

Caregivers often find apathy especially painful because it can feel like the person they love no longer cares. In reality, the ability to initiate or express engagement may be impaired even when emotional connection remains.

Caregiver Burnout

Physical, emotional, and mental exhaustion caused by prolonged caregiving stress. Symptoms may include fatigue, irritability, anxiety, depression, and feeling overwhelmed or detached.

Dementia

An umbrella term describing a group of symptoms caused by changes in the brain that affect memory, thinking, behavior, communication, and daily functioning. Dementia is progressive and varies widely between individuals.

Hospice

A form of care focused on comfort, dignity, and quality of life rather than cure. Hospice supports both the person nearing the end of life and their caregivers through medical, emotional, and practical care.

HIPAA Authorization

A legal document that allows healthcare providers to share medical information with designated individuals. Without it, caregivers may be excluded from medical discussions.

Incontinence

Loss of bladder or bowel control. In dementia, this is typically caused by neurological changes rather than behavioral choice.

Long-Term Care Insurance

An insurance policy that may help cover costs associated with long-term care, such as in-home care, memory care, or skilled nursing. Coverage varies widely by policy.

Memory Care

A specialized type of residential care designed for individuals with dementia. These facilities provide structured routines, trained staff, and enhanced safety measures.

Medicaid

A government program that may cover long-term care for individuals who meet medical and financial eligibility requirements. Medicaid coverage and availability vary by state.

Medicare

A federal health insurance program for people over 65 or with certain disabilities. Medicare does **not** cover long-term custodial care.

Palliative Care (Comfort Care)

A form of supportive care focused on comfort, quality of life, and relief from distress for people living with serious or long-term illness. Palliative care can begin early in the disease process and may be provided alongside other treatments. It supports both the individual and their caregivers by addressing physical symptoms, emotional needs, and overall well-being — with an emphasis on dignity and comfort.

Palliative Care vs. Hospice Care

Palliative care supports comfort and quality of life throughout serious illness, while hospice care is specifically designed for the final stage of life when the focus is entirely on comfort rather than cure.

Power of Attorney (Financial)

A legal document that allows someone to manage another person's financial matters when the other person is unable to do so safely.

Healthcare Power of Attorney

A legal document that designates someone to make medical decisions if a person becomes unable to communicate or understand their care options.

Sundowning

A pattern in which confusion, anxiety, agitation, or restlessness increases in the late afternoon or evening. Sundowning is common in dementia but varies in severity.

UTI (Urinary Tract Infection)

An infection that can cause sudden confusion, agitation, or behavioral changes in people with dementia. UTIs may present without typical symptoms like pain or fever.

Vascular Dementia

A type of dementia caused by reduced blood flow to the brain, often following strokes or vascular disease. Symptoms may appear suddenly or progress unevenly.

A Final Note on Language

Language around dementia can feel cold or clinical. These terms exist to help communicate—not to define your loved one or your experience.

You are not required to use perfect language to be a good caregiver.

Understanding grows over time—and compassion matters more than terminology.

Appendix B — Resources for Caregivers and Grief Support

You are not meant to do this alone.

These resources are here to support you—whether you are caregiving, considering placement, navigating hospice, or grieving a loss.

You don't need to contact all of them. Seek out the one(s) that resonate with your journey.

Dementia-Specific Support

Alzheimer's Association

Website: alz.org

Helpline (U.S.): 1-800-272-3900 (24/7)

- Education about all types of dementia (not only Alzheimer's)
- Caregiver support groups (online and local)
- A 24/7 helpline staffed by trained professionals
- Help navigating diagnosis, care options, and next steps

This is often the most comprehensive starting point for caregivers.

Teepa Snow's Positive Approach to Care

https://www.youtube.com/@teepasnowvideos

Caregiver Support & Aging Services

Area Agency on Aging (AAA)

Access: eldercare.acl.gov (U.S.)

- Connects caregivers to local resources
- Help with respite care, transportation, meals, and benefits
- Guidance on Medicaid, long-term care options, and services

Search by ZIP code to find your local agency.

Book Resources (available on Amazon.com)

- *Contented Dementia* by Oliver James
- *Learning to Speak Alzheimer's* by Joanne Koenig Coste
- *The 36-Hour Day* by Nancy L. Mace & Peter V. Rabins
- *The Dementia Caregiver's Survival Guide* by Linda S. Erwin

Facebook Groups

There are a huge amount of groups dedicated to dementia and caregiving on Facebook. Listed below are the three I frequent the most.

- Alzheimer's/Dementia Help & Support Group - https://www.facebook.com/groups/394602195862976
- Dementia/Alzheimers Family Caregiver Support - https://www.facebook.com/groups/1490883851158632

- Speaking Dementia -
  https://www.facebook.com/profile.php?id=6155837692
  0257

Family Caregiver Alliance

Website: caregiver.org

- Caregiver education and support
- Articles on burnout, boundaries, and self-care
- Support for caregivers across diagnoses

Hospice & End-of-Life Support

National Hospice and Palliative Care Organization

Website: nhpco.org

- Education about hospice and palliative care
- Help finding hospice providers
- Guidance for families navigating end-of-life decisions

Hospice support is for caregivers too—not just patients.

Mental Health & Crisis Support

988 Suicide & Crisis Lifeline

Call or Text: 988 (U.S., 24/7)

- Free, confidential support

- For moments of emotional overwhelm, despair, or crisis
- You do not need to be suicidal to call

If you feel unsafe or at the end of your rope, please reach out.

Outside the U.S.:

Visit local health services websites or search "suicide crisis hotline" with your country name for immediate support options.

Grief and Bereavement Support

GriefShare

Website: griefshare.org

- Structured grief support groups (often faith-based)
- In-person and online options
- Useful for people who prefer guided group support

Local Hospice Bereavement Programs

Many hospice organizations offer **free grief counseling or support groups** for months after a death—even if your loved one did not receive hospice care through them.

Call local hospice providers and ask about bereavement services.

Legal and Financial Guidance

- **Elder law attorneys** (for power of attorney, guardianship, Medicaid planning)

- **Legal aid organizations** (often available for low-income families)
- **Social workers** through hospitals, clinics, or hospice agencies

Ask providers directly for referrals—many caregivers don't realize this help is available.

A Final Word About Asking for Help

Needing help does not mean you failed.

Feeling overwhelmed does not mean you're weak.

Reaching out does not mean you gave up.

Caregiving and grief are not meant to be endured in isolation.

Support is part of care.

With Gratitude

This book exists because of the people who were willing to walk beside me — and to speak honestly about an experience that is so often carried in silence.

I am deeply grateful to the people in my life who read the first manuscript of this book and shared their stories, reflections, and hard-earned wisdom. Your feedback helped shape this work in ways that truly mattered.

Thank you to **Cathy Wohlk, Chrysty Fortner, Debbie Pole, Elizabeth Sabiston, Doug Reinhardt, Joanne Welling, Joan Metz, and Dianne Denny**.

Thank you to those who trusted me with their lived experience, their vulnerability, and their time. Dementia caregiving can feel isolating, and your openness helped ensure this book would not be written from theory alone, but from shared reality.

And to my mom — who continues to teach me about presence, resilience, and love in forms I never expected — this book is shaped by our journey together. **Bertie, you are still a force.**

Thank you to **Tony and Cathy Santore** for walking alongside me during my darkest times, for never saying "just move past it" or "maybe if you stop talking about it, it will get better." Thank you for your love, your steadiness, and for sharing your family and puppies.

Thank you to **Pam Karabatsos** for being my "always." There aren't words...

Any remaining shortcomings in this book are mine alone.

A Final Note to You

If you've reached the end of this book, I want to pause with you for a moment.

Reading this far says something important: you have been living inside something incredibly hard. Whether you are at the beginning of this journey, deep in the middle, or finding your way through what comes after, you didn't pick this path — but you've been walking it with courage.

Dementia caregiving asks more of people than most will ever understand. It asks for patience when there is no clarity, strength when there is no rest, and love that keeps adapting as loss unfolds in pieces. It asks you to make decisions without certainty, to carry grief while still functioning, and to keep showing up even when the person you love cannot meet you where they once did.

If there were moments in this book that felt too close to home, too heavy, or too familiar, I hope you also felt less alone reading them. That was always my intention.

I want you to hear this clearly:

You did not imagine how hard this was.
You were not weak for feeling overwhelmed.
You were not wrong for needing help.

There is no perfect way to care for someone with dementia. There are only thoughtful, loving choices made under impossible circumstances. And those choices — even the ones that still ache — came from care.

If you are still caregiving, I hope you continue to give yourself permission to rest, to ask for help, and to adjust as things change. If caregiving has ended, I hope you are gentle with yourself as you grieve not only your loved one, but the version of yourself shaped by years of responsibility.

The love you gave did not disappear when memory faded.
The care you offered mattered — even when it felt invisible.

Whatever comes next for you, I hope you carry this with you: you showed up. Again and again. In ways that counted.

Thank you for trusting me with your time, your story, and your heart.

You are not alone.

— *Sheri Rettew*

P.S. I hope you'll meet me at www.dementiacaregroup.com and continue the conversation for yourself and for all of the caregivers of the world.